A[DVICE]

from a

PREGNANT
OBSTETRICIAN

ADVICE
from a
PREGNANT OBSTETRICIAN

An Insider's Guide

SHARI BRASNER, M.D.

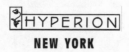

NEW YORK

The information imparted in this book is comprised of the medical knowledge, personal experience, and, in many instances, the
opinions of its author. This is merely one doctor's view, and
none of the issues addressed in the book should replace the
advice given to a woman by her own obstetrician.

Library of Congress Cataloging-in-Publication Data

Brasner, Shari.
  Advice from a pregnant obstetrician: an insider's guide /
Shari Brasner.—1st ed.
    p.   cm.
  ISBN: 0-7868-8339-1
  1. Pregnancy. 2. Childbirth. I. Title.
RG525.B662 1998
618.2'4—dc21   97-36475
                                                CIP

Book design by Christine Weathersbee

FIRST EDITION

10 9 8 7 6 5 4 3 2 1

This book is dedicated to my children, Samantha and Zachary, who bring me joy every day. My husband, Jeffrey Cohen, has unconditionally supported me as both physician and mother.

I thank my colleagues in private practice, Drs. Austin Abramson, Karen Brodman, and Lynn Friedman, for serving as role models. They continue to teach me the art of combining good medical judgment with good bedside manner.

I thank my editor, Jennifer Barth, whose eye for detail helped shape this book.

And finally, I thank Richard Panek, who shared his time and editorial wisdom, and Meg Wolitzer, for her inspiration. They have become special friends and made the whole effort an enjoyable learning experience.

contents

first trimester

It was a fairly common occurrence for me, back during my first pregnancy, to wake up in the middle of the night, startled into consciousness not so much by the pressure of a full bladder (although that was part of it) as by the fear that I had done something wrong, something that would make the baby growing inside me turn out to be less than perfect. You have to understand that a lot of this is simply who I am: part hypochondriac, part guilt-ridden individual for reasons I haven't yet uncovered during the psychoanalytic hour, and part lover of all things dramatic. But many of my middle-of-the-night fears and preoccupations were the sort of fears and preoccupations shared by other pregnant women I knew.

I would lie awake in bed and count out the grams of protein I had eaten that day, or else obsess over the single tranquilizer I had taken before I knew I was pregnant. Sometimes I would squint in the darkened bedroom at the expanding hill that was my stomach, and I would think that it looked a little too small for where I was in my pregnancy—perhaps I would eventually give birth to a teensy baby, roughly the size of a sock puppet. Occasionally, in the middle of this reverie of self-flagellation and misery, I would even begin to cry quietly, and my husband would wake up and ask me what was wrong.

"I've done something terrible," I'd say, regaling him with stories of how I had wolfed down an actual Kit-Kat bar that afternoon, a treat that was made up entirely of useless, potentially harmful sugar. I would even try to include him as an accessory to a crime: "Remember that night a few months ago?" I'd say to him in the dark. "We were downtown and it was raining, and you wanted to stop in at Fanelli's, so I said okay? And then I ordered a drink at the bar! And it turned out I was pregnant and didn't know it yet, and it was your idea that we go to Fanelli's in the first place!"

My attempt to draw him into the guilt over what, I was now convinced, would be a terrible pregnancy outcome, was never successful. He feared neither the pregnancy nor its result. He was happy to keep bopping along each day, accompanying me to the occasional obstetrical visit to listen to the fetal heartbeat, or sitting cross-legged on the floor at childbirth class, or sometimes chatting lightly with me about middle names for the baby. But he refused to indulge me in what he considered my ridiculous, and ridiculously pessimistic, thinking. That I had to do alone, and do it I did, usually in the middle of the night.

Sometimes it wasn't fear that awakened me, but nagging questions which I had never thought to address with my obstetrician, or hadn't yet had the chance to ask. Occasionally in the early months, I would try to entrap my husband into a debate over whether or not I should undergo an amniocentesis, even though I was only 31 at the time. I would attempt to coax him into a feverish middle-of-the-night discussion that included all the amnio pros and cons I'd managed to come up with. If anything happened to the baby because I'd decided to have an amnio, I told him, I'd never *forgive* myself. On the other hand, wasn't it better to know the baby's genetic makeup, and be as completely informed as possible?

"Are you just about finished?" he'd ask me finally, and I would say yes, I was.

He would stare at me for a long moment, telling me how sad it was that our child was going to be raised by a truly insane mother. And then he would turn over and go back to sleep.

I, however, would lie awake for quite some time.

When I look back on those difficult, sleepless nights of my first pregnancy, I now feel enough distance from them to transform all the anxiety I experienced into a slew of funny little anecdotes about one pregnant woman's idiosyncratic neuroses. (Which could make up a book of their own, shelved in bookstores under "Pregnancy," "Humor," and "Abnormal Psychology.") But really, at the time it was happening, I felt absolutely no ironic detachment at all. I was pregnant and very glad to be, but I was also scared of what was happening to me: scared of what I'd already done, and what awaited me in the future.

To paraphrase Butterfly McQueen, I didn't know nothing about birthing no baby.

I'd assumed, initially, that reading books would help. Most of us, raised to love and trust books, seek them out whenever there's a new topic that we know little about. I went to the bookstore the day I took the home pregnancy stick test and the second blue line unequivocally appeared. There, newly pregnant and trembling with the excitement and novelty of the news, I stationed myself not in the usual "Recent Fiction" section, but instead in the "Pregnancy and Child-Care" corner, which was quite full to bursting, as I myself would be soon enough. There were guidebooks and reference books and books that told you what to eat (all the recipes seemed to include either rolled oats or bran flakes), and there was a book with alarmingly vivid photographs of a growing fetus. I armed myself with several of these books in the hope that at least one of them would both educate and calm me.

Unfortunately, I found that no book could do both. Some books assumed a rather stern, authoritative, guilt-inducing tone, which I'm convinced eventually helped lead to my middle-of-the-night panic. Others were so laid-back and calm in a "just take it easy and it will all be fine" way, that I just knew they were hiding something; it was as though the authors felt pregnant women were fragile creatures who couldn't tolerate being told the truth. And still others disseminated information without being accusatory, yet they also spread all the facts out in front of the reader without any bias whatsoever, objectively describing various options in pregnancy, such as amnio vs. CVS, or epidurals vs. drug-free childbirth. Faced with this huge catalog of sophisticated medical decisions, pregnant women were supposed to choose for themselves what kinds of tests and pain relief they wanted. This wasn't like picking a dress to wear to a party, or deciding which movie to go to at the sixplex. This was about something truly important. How could I, a total novice, possibly know what to do?

Enter *Advice from a Pregnant Obstetrician*, the first book that aims to give the reader all the necessary information a pregnant woman needs in a voice of empathy, common sense, and experience—both personal and professional. What the reader is going through, Dr. Brasner has already gone through. This is the only book I know of to offer an array of actual opinions—telling you what the doctor did when she was in your shoes (and why), as well as exactly what she tells her patients when they come to her with the same fears, questions, and real medical concerns. She takes the pregnant reader through every step of the three trimesters, explaining things that a woman might feel her own obstetrician was too busy to talk about in depth. Perhaps, after reading Shari Brasner's words, you will think, as I do now, that I'd been too hard on myself when I was pregnant for the first time.

But I didn't have *Advice from a Pregnant Obstetrician* back then to help me separate anxiety from reality, and to guide me through a maze that included everything from the most important life-altering decisions to the most annoying symptoms. Instead, I had a shelf full of books beside my bed that offered a great deal of confusing information, and then backed away from responsibility by adding the caveat, "Your doctor, of course, will be your primary source of information." Of course, that is true—no book can ever replace a doctor, nor should it try. But all too often, doctors aren't helpful enough when it comes time for a woman to figure out how to feel or what to do about certain matters. It may not be that the doctors are too neutral, but that their waiting rooms are simply too busy to allow for a great deal of hand-holding, but even so, it can leave a woman feeling very confused.

Pregnancy can be a time in which level-headed decision-making can easily be swept away under the tide of emotion that women often experience. I remember being embarrassed to admit to feeling so weepy and excited and forgetful; it seemed almost sexist to think that pregnancy could do this to me. I had the idea that I ought to keep this information to myself, lest it fall into the wrong hands. ("You see?" I could almost hear a voice saying. "That's why women can never be president. They're ruled by their hormones!")

Then there were the dreams. Most of the pregnant women I know have had peculiar, and peculiarly vivid, dreams about the impending birth. For me, the most frequently appearing dream was one that I came to call "The Lost Baby." In the dream, I've just given birth to a newborn about as big as a peanut and made of wax, and I make a nice little crib for the baby, place him in it, leave the room, and . . . promptly forget where I put him. Then I find myself frantically searching the house for my poor little wax baby, but I never do find him. I would usually wake up from this dream glazed with sweat, thinking, *Poor baby! Poor me! I'm not cut out for this at all!*

My second pregnancy, I should add, was a whole different ball game: an easy game of catch, as opposed to the first pregnancy's elaborate and highly technical game of *baccie* conducted entirely in a foreign language. By the time I became pregnant with my younger son, I had no desire to read a single pregnancy book, or even obsess much about being pregnant. I realized, to my surprise, that I was actually calm this time around. I had very few weird dreams, and only an occasional strange anxiety. Once in a while, though, I still looked through the pregnant woman's metaphorical window, in which the shape of her life changes before her—and I was still amazed.

The truth is, once you have gone through pregnancy, you will never forget anything about it. It is an experience that changes and instructs and thrills you, even while keeping you up in the middle of the night, plagued with worries that are not only unnecessary but also probably silly. But it's the rare woman who goes through the experience without at least a few bad dreams, minor freak-outs, or moments of self-flagellation.

No one I know thinks she was "cut out" to be a mother, and yet our reproductive organs tell a different story entirely. They're working, functioning, fusing sperm and egg, spinning rapidly, and creating this amazing growing thing that one day we will call a baby. No matter how inadequate we may feel, or how much we may worry that we've been negligent or cavalier or destructive, the body knows better, and keeps doing what it does best.

Now that I'm no longer pregnant, and probably won't ever go through pregnancy again, I have to say that in a peculiar way I actually miss those sleepless, wired, obsessive nights, those alternately jittery and thrilled days. If I'd had Shari Brasner's book back then, I would probably have gotten more sleep and frittered away less time in pointless worry. If I'd had someone to offer informed opinions and explain why she—a doctor and former pregnant woman— thinks and feels the way she does about a host of issues that were relevant to me, then maybe I could have relaxed a little bit more and enjoyed the show.

And what a show it is. The first heartbeat, the first kick, the last push: I still remember them all. By the way, the little lost wax baby of my strange pregnancy dreams is now seven years old, loves Scooby-Doo cartoons and basketball, and has his mother's eyes.

Long before I became pregnant with my twins, Zachary and Samantha, I thought I knew everything I needed to know about pregnancy. After all, I'd been an obstetrician for years, and I'd already delivered hundreds and hundreds of babies. I liked to think of myself as a competent, caring doctor—someone young and casual, someone you could really talk to. And women did talk to me: Whether pregnant or trying to get pregnant, they came into my office and asked volumes of questions, which I happily answered. This was my job, after all, and I'd always loved it. I tried to give patients all the time and attention I could spare, even though I often had a waiting room populated by other pregnant women who had their own questions to ask. In short, I thought I was doing a pretty decent job helping to shepherd pregnant women through the most intensely thrilling and potentially nerve-racking nine months of their lives.

And then I became pregnant myself.

While the twins grew and developed and thrashed around inside me, I received a crash course in obstetrics that no medical school textbook or residency ever could have provided. Having been pregnant has absolutely made me a better doctor, and it's also made me want to write a book that gives pregnant women the inside track on everything they need to know during the coming months. I'm aware that there are plenty of other pregnancy guides out there; I've listened to nervous patients recite whole sections almost word for word, and I consulted several such books during my own pregnancy. But this book, I hope, has something more, something no other guide of this type offers: the essential view from both sides of the stirrups.

This book is a labor of love from someone who not only has cared for pregnant women and caught their babies, but also has felt the gallop of feet (four at once) inside her own body. As a formerly pregnant woman, I know what you *want* to know. As a currently practicing obstetrician, I know what you *need* to know. I've tried to make this book comprehensive yet clear, and how I've done that is by eliminating the mixed signals that other guides so often seem to give. Pregnancy can be a confusing enough time without having a book overwhelm you with sterile information and on-the-one-hand/on-the-other-hand alternatives. If I know something, you'll know it; if I have an opinion, you'll hear it.

And that's probably what most separates this book from the pack of pregnancy guides out there: me. It simply might not be possible for you to ask your obstetrician about every last one of the topics covered in the next couple of hundred pages. Even the kindest, most patient, most generous doctor probably has other patients, or a home to go to.

Not me. I'm all yours. For once in your life, you have the undivided attention of a doctor. I'm not really your obstetrician, but I play that role in this book. And here, in the cozy office of the blank page, where the chairs are always leather, the unseen radio plays commercial-free classical, and even the magazines out in the waiting room are fresh, you and I have all the time in the world. The phone is off the hook, my beeper is out of batteries.

So go ahead. Ask me anything.

ADVICE
from a
PREGNANT
OBSTETRICIAN

the *first*
trimester

 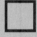

Chapter One

Baby Steps

- Confirming the Pregnancy
- Choosing a Doctor
- Scheduling the First Visit

When a pregnant woman comes to see an obstetrician for the first time, she's often slightly giddy with expectation—pun intended—and often slightly freaked out as well. After all, the state of being pregnant today is very different from what it was in our mothers' era. In those days, women were expected not to ask questions of their doctors, but to loll around looking pretty in shapeless garments for nine months, drinking malteds, and shopping for wallpaper. When they went to the obstetrician, he was often a paternal, chuckling, silver-haired figure who told women to "relax" and kept them in the dark about many of the details of their own pregnancies. Back then, very few women questioned these methods, and the pregnancy progressed like some weird underground event.

Those days are gone. The women I see in my practice want information about their pregnancies—and the more information, the better. These are women who, presumably like you, want to understand what's going on inside their bodies, and want to know what sorts of changes and tests and decisions will take place over the coming months. They don't want to be condescended to by doctors. These are *their* bodies, *their* pregnancies. They want to know what's happening at each obstetrical visit: when to pay close attention, when to worry a little, and when, most importantly, to relax.

One of the biggest mistakes women make during pregnancy is to view their condition as an illness. They think, *If I need to see a doctor, I must be sick.* Let me emphasize right here, at the start, that this is definitely *not* the way obstetricians see it. Pregnancy is not a disease; it's a normal part of life. I always make sure my patients realize this, and when I was pregnant myself I felt better than ever for much of the time. It's a great boost for the baby to have a mother who's been paying attention to the details. While you don't need to be an M.D. yourself to go through a successful pregnancy, I think it's helpful to start these months armed with a good attitude and plenty of sound advice.

CONFIRMING THE PREGNANCY

The first step is the obvious one: making sure. Many people won't believe the results of a home pregnancy test until it's confirmed by a doctor—even if the home pregnancy test is emitting a blindingly pink positive sign. They'll take a test again, and again, and yet again, until they've spent $50 or more and used test sticks are cluttering the bathroom counter.

In fact, these tests have a 99 percent rate of accuracy, as they claim on the side of the package. Sometimes women

won't believe the result until the test is done again in the
doctor's office, but our urine tests have the same sensitivity
as the type you buy in a drugstore. (The kind of meaningful
testing we can offer that you *can't* buy in a drugstore is a
blood test, which is, medically speaking, quite useful, but
more on that later.) What's more, when the instructions on
a home pregnancy test say that even the faintest indication
of a positive result should be interpreted as, indeed, a positive result, they mean it. This is not to say that mistakes
never happen; but they don't happen nearly often enough
to merit a third and fourth home test or the needless anxiety that goes with them.

Once you've confirmed your pregnancy, that's the time
to think about:

CHOOSING A DOCTOR

Many women choose as their obstetrician the doctor who
for years has served as their gynecologist. But some women
don't have that choice. Their gynecologists aren't obstetricians, or perhaps they simply think it's time to start fresh.
After all, it can be a pretty big leap to think of the doctor
who twice a year wields a Pap smear swab or fits you for a
diaphragm as the same person who will walk you through
the variously astonishing or dizzying stages of pregnancy
and, at the end of it all, tenderly and safely deliver your
baby. As the old expression goes, "A Pap smear is only a
Pap smear, but a baby is a *baby*." (All right, there's no such
expression, but there should be.)

In choosing an obstetrician, you should consider the following criteria, which I myself kept in mind while making
my choice. (No, I didn't stay with my partners in my own

practice; that would have been too much like asking a member of my family to treat me.) Even if you're leaning toward staying with your gynecologist, I would still urge you to review these considerations.

• **Size of the practice.** These days, it's less common to find an obstetrician practicing on his or her own, but lone baby-catchers still do exist. One of the advantages to choosing a solo practitioner is that you can forge a strong bond with him or her and not be burdened by the conflicting information that you might receive from the different doctors in a group practice. But when I chose a doctor, I opted for a group practice because I knew that solo practitioners often have to reschedule appointments due to unexpected deliveries and emergencies. I also knew that when it came time for my twins to shove off, there was a decent chance my doctor would be on vacation or delivering someone else. When your own doctor isn't available, then you may be left with a covering doctor, someone you might not know at all, and possibly someone you might not like very much.

For all these reasons, I chose a two-person practice where the partners covered only for each other, and I made sure that I liked both doctors. I considered myself a patient of both doctors, and I strongly recommend that you do the same. In my own practice, my three partners and I trade off being on call on weekends and nights. We also encourage patients to make the first two appointments with the same doctor, then rotate among us. We get to know all of our obstetrical patients, as any one of us might deliver her when the time comes.

• **The hospital with which the doctor is affiliated.** You may wonder, How does someone "choose" a hospital? No one *likes* them, not the way people might like a restaurant or a movie. They're basically big, scary, impersonal places that smell of disinfectant. Don't be fooled by hospitals that appear small and intimate and are filled with potted plants. Don't choose a hospital by the food, or according to whether it has a park view. Those are all excellent criteria for a bed-and-breakfast, but not necessarily for a facility that's expert in the practice of medicine. You want a first-rate hospital. Find out the following three things:

1. *Is the hospital a teaching hospital?*

2. *Does it have a neonatal intensive care unit capable of handling a premature delivery or a serious medical condition?*

3. *Is there a full-time anesthesiology staff assigned to labor and delivery on the obstetrical unit?*

While right now you may be thinking only about yourself and your pregnancy, there will be a baby some months down the line. Most babies are perfect, but some do need extra help, so you need to be sure your hospital has the appropriate high-tech support services. This means that ideally you want what is known as a "teaching" hospital, where seasoned doctors teach residents and interns—a place that's affiliated with a university or medical school, that's involved in research, that's well versed in the latest techniques. It also means that there are always obstetricians and pediatricians in-house all night long in case you or your baby has a problem and your doctor isn't present.

My practice is located in New York City, where there is no shortage of major teaching hospitals with neonatal intensive care units. But if you live in a small town or rural area, the question may arise as to whether it's worth making the trek (sometimes even 100 miles away) to a better, more high-powered facility, or whether it's acceptable to have the baby at a much more convenient, less "presti-gious" place. This is a personal decision, of course, that may involve extra expenses and the inconvenience of hav-ing to travel a long way for ultrasounds, testing, and deliv-ery. But I find that the same question arises even in New York City, when patients from the outlying area must decide whether to choose an obstetrician affiliated with a first-rate hospital in Manhattan. In our practice, we have plenty of patients who regularly drive an hour and a half or longer for their obstetrical visits because they feel that the level of care they're going to get at our hospital is signifi-cantly better than what's available locally, especially in the event of an emergency.

Some women worry that they live so far away that when they go into labor they're not going to make it to the hospi-tal in time. For the most part, I can reassure these women that things tend not to happen all that quickly, especially in a first pregnancy. Once in a while, though—less often than you might think—the progress of labor is surprisingly rapid, and if this happens I will send a woman to a hospital close to her home rather than have her risk a long trip and the possibility of getting stuck in traffic.

The issue of anesthesia is also worth considering. While most large teaching hospitals have their own full-time anes-thesia staff, some smaller, non-teaching hospitals don't. Instead, they have individual contracts with anesthesiolo-gists who agree to come in when you're in labor. I'm not in favor of this idea, because it means you may have to wait in excruciating pain to get your epidural or delay an emer-gency cesarean until an anesthesiologist finally arrives. Don't be shy; ask your doctor what the policy is at the hospi-tal where you'll be delivering.

• **Availability.** Of course you want a terrific, sensitive, smart, experienced doctor, but what good are those qualities if you can't have access to them for weeks at a time? It might mean that this doctor is popular—the warmest, youngest, most stylish Armani-clad female obstetrician around, whom all your friends adore—but it also might mean that her office isn't as flexible as it ought to be. How can you find out in advance if your obstetrician will "be there for you"?

1. *Office hours.* Look for an office where the doctors are willing to stay late or come in a little early to squeeze in appointments with new OB patients or to accommodate a working woman's schedule. If hours start before 9:00 A.M. and extend past 5:00 P.M., that's a good indication of the office's philosophy about flexibility.

2. *Find out if pregnant patients get priority.* To a doctor in my line of work, a phone call from a 50-year-old woman with a vaginal itch shouldn't carry the same urgency as a call from a pregnant woman who's worried about spotting or unusual pain. As I've said, pregnancy isn't an illness, but an obstetrician should never forget that there's a new life forming in there—and if that's not enough to get a doctor to pick up the phone and return a call, then I don't know what is.

• **Your own gut reaction.** It's not a scientific phenomenon, it's not a medical consideration, but it should definitely be a factor in choosing an obstetrician. To some extent, all the considerations I've listed above are matters of personal taste, but others are even more individualistic. It's hard for a patient to choose an obstetrician based on medical "philosophies," and I can't really think of any meaningful questions you could ask a doctor about his or her practice of obstetrics, except perhaps one: What is the practice's cesarean section rate? The national average hovers at around 25 percent, so if this doctor quotes a number higher than that, I would probably investigate further. Cesarean section is a surgical procedure that one would hope to avoid unless it is medically indicated. There are doctors who sometimes perform C-sections to hasten delivery and accommodate their schedules. Don't assume, however, that a number slightly higher than 25 percent means that a doctor is acting solely in his or her own interest. Does the doctor specialize in high-risk pregnancies? Does the doctor utilize the modern technologies that help assess fetal status in labor, such as fetal scalp sampling? Does he or she believe in vaginal delivery after a previous cesarean? Getting this sort of information might help elucidate what may seem to be an excessively high number.

Here are a few questions you might want to use as a guideline when meeting with a new obstetrician, or even if you're deciding whether to stay with your old gynecologist.

1. *Do I feel completely comfortable with this doctor?* Comfortable enough to be able to ask any questions that I want to, without being made to feel embarrassed or dumb? (And this includes potentially squeamish matters such as sexually-transmitted diseases, weird fears, etc.)

2. *Is this a person I can tolerate having fairly regular contact with—meaning a dozen or more visits— over the better part of a year?*

3. Will I feel okay having to call this person in the middle of the night, if need be?

4. Is this someone who makes time to talk to me, and who, although very busy, runs his or her office with calm and empathy, and not with factory-like impersonality?

If you've answered "no" to any of the above, you should at least consider another doctor. Now is the time to find someone you like and trust. You don't have to believe that this person will be your best friend forever, but you will have to feel comfortable discussing a host of intimate issues with this person for months to come.

SCHEDULING THE FIRST VISIT

Finding a doctor, of course, is only half the task. Now comes the question of when to see your doctor for the first time. The receptionist will often help a patient calculate how many weeks it's been since her last menstrual period, and schedule the first visit accordingly. In my practice, we want to see women on the early side, not just to be kind or hand-holdingly cozy, but for medical reasons. Such as:

• **To confirm the pregnancy.** As I mentioned, some women won't believe the news until a doctor has confirmed it. As a result, they might not only be subjecting themselves to unnecessary anxiety, but, more importantly, they might not be taking proper care of themselves until the news feels "real."

• **To date the pregnancy.** The earlier we confirm the pregnancy and establish viability, the better we are at gestational dating, which will become important later on. Many women are surprised by the date I give them, even when their menstrual history has seemed reliable. (For a full explanation of how we date a pregnancy, see page 16.)

• **To rule out undetected life-threatening emergencies,** such as an ectopic pregnancy. The word "ectopic" refers to something that's "in the wrong place." The most common "wrong place" that ectopic pregnancies occur is the fallopian tubes. The fertilized egg attaches itself to a tube, as opposed to the lining of the uterus. Very occasionally we even see a fertilized egg attach itself to the abdomen or to an ovary. The danger in an ectopic pregnancy is that the structure to which the egg has attached itself is not equipped to accommodate a growing embryo, and could become damaged, creating a true emergency. A fallopian tube, for instance, could rupture and hemorrhage. The earlier we can make the diagnosis, the less risk there might be to the patient. If we were to discover an ectopic pregnancy in its early stages, for example, we might be able simply to cut open the tube and let it heal, as opposed to removing the tube entirely.

I suggest that the best time to schedule a first appointment is about six to seven weeks from the last menstrual period (LMP), or about two to three weeks after a missed period. But I'm happy to see a woman who's gotten a positive result from a home pregnancy test even one day after her missed period. I'm limited in my ability to assess the health of her pregnancy at that stage, but I can still start to convey important information. This may be especially important to a woman with a history of ectopic pregnancy, miscarriage, or other poor outcomes.

And if the nurse or receptionist tries to block you from coming in before some mythical eight-week period has passed, you might want to reconsider your choice of an obstetrical office. After all, you'll be dealing with the front-desk people in your doctor's office fairly often over the course of your pregnancy, and you can get a good sense from this initial interaction as to how you'll be treated. If the receptionist is like a lion at the gate, unyielding and a bit ferocious, and she won't check with the doctor to see if "rules" can be bent, then this may indicate what the entire experience with this office will be like—snappish, or stand-offish, or at least bound to make you feel like a hypochondriac whenever you call with a question.

My partners and I, as I've mentioned, encourage the patient to make the first two appointments with the same doctor in our group, then rotate and get to know everyone. The first two visits are the ones in which most of the meat and bones of pregnancy are covered, and we feel that if this initial information is offered in one voice it might be easier for the patient to process. Also, this helps reassure the patient that the information is complete.

This is what the chronology of visits for a routine pregnancy typically looks like in our practice:

• Once we establish a healthy pregnancy, around the eight-week mark, we'll see a patient every four weeks or so until:

• 24 weeks. At this point we'll see a patient every three weeks, until:

• 32 weeks. Now we'll want to see a patient every other week, until:

• 36 weeks. This is the home stretch, when visits increase to once a week, until:

• Delivery. From the doctor's point of view, after the information-gathering and -disseminating of the first couple of visits, most of the rest of the appointments are little more than checkups—important, to be sure, and often reassuring for both patient and doctor, but routine checkups nonetheless. And as long as they stay routine, there's little to worry about.

But there's plenty to learn, if you're the patient, especially a first-timer. In a way, part of the point of this book is to provide you with a doctor's perspective on what a routine pregnancy is, how to keep it routine, and what you can do if it turns out not to be routine. Remember, though, that very few pregnancies turn out to be predictable in every last detail. But we're getting ahead of ourselves. It's a long way from now until the day your baby is born—dozens of weeks, several months, and, to be absolutely precise about it, eight chapters, away.

Chapter Two

The New You

- Dating the Pregnancy
- Blood Pressure, Urine, and Blood
- Physical Changes
- Feeling Bad Physically
- Feeling Bad Emotionally
- Illnesses
- Risk or Fear of Miscarriage
- Genetic Testing
- Chorionic Villus Sampling
- First-Trimester Bleeding
- Multiple Fetuses
- Preexisting Medical Conditions

So there you are, sitting in the office of the doctor you've chosen. You've gotten over the novelty of being pregnant, the initial thrill or jolt as well as the first important decision about which doctor is going to deliver your baby. You're ready to move on to the nuts and bolts of pregnancy, both the small issues and the larger ones.

For a first visit, I devote at least a half hour to taking a personal history, performing a full physical exam including a pelvic, and then opening the floor to questions. Often I will run over by ten minutes or so. (Think about this the next time you're kept seething, flipping through shopworn copies of *People* in a waiting room: Maybe your doctor is particularly generous with her time, and soon you'll reap those benefits, too.) While in the next couple of chapters I will focus on *your* particular concerns at this time—the endless list that most pregnant women unfurl in front of their doctors like some ancient scroll—I think it might help you put this information into perspective if I first explain, in this chapter, what I as a doctor am thinking about and focusing on when you come into my office newly pregnant.

DATING THE PREGNANCY

Obstetricians date a pregnancy from the first day of the last menstrual period, or LMP. We call a due date the EDC, which are the initials for the very Victorian-sounding "estimated date of confinement." The EDC is established using something called Naegle's Rule. What you do is this: Subtract three months from the LMP, then add one week, and that's your due date. You'll see your doctor pull out a little wheel and turn it, matching up dates in order to find out when you're due. That wheel, which is a circular calendar, is the closest measure we have, but sometimes you'll find that your friends or your mother calculated your due date and came up with an entirely different date. That's because your doctor counts in weeks from the LMP, and your friends count in months, and the two systems don't always correlate—especially if your friends make the common mistake of figuring a month as four weeks, instead of the four-and-a-fraction it actually is.

For the record: Full term is 40 weeks, or about nine months plus one week.

When I ask a new patient to tell me the date of her LMP, it's good information to get from her, but it's not crucial. Women can be wrong (or completely clueless) about the date, so in my practice, we like to corroborate it with an ultrasound (also known as a sonogram). The earlier the peek, the more accurately we can date the pregnancy. (That's our preference, but if it's not an option your doctor offers, that's perfectly acceptable. For more about ultrasounds, see page 97.) Also, I've had patients who were wildly off in terms of how pregnant they thought they were, because what they thought of as their LMP was, in fact, something called implantation bleeding, which can happen at the very start of a pregnancy. (For more on implantation bleeding, see page 41.) During the entire time of their supposed "period," they were, in fact, pregnant, and their babies were therefore due four or six weeks earlier than they expected.

In our practice, we give each patient her own wheel at the first visit, and you might ask your doctor if you can have one, too. I find that, at a point in the pregnancy when the whole experience is somewhat disorienting and abstract, the little gift of a wheel can help the patient to think of her pregnancy in more concrete terms; it literally gives her something to hold on to.

BLOOD PRESSURE, URINE, AND BLOOD

At the first visit, in addition to performing a full physical exam, checking thyroid, breasts, abdomen, pelvis, and a

Pap smear, the obstetrician will perform several simple tests. These include blood pressure, a urine sample, and a blood sample, and we do them for the following reasons:

• **Blood pressure.** The doctor takes the pregnant patient's blood pressure at the first appointment for two reasons: to make sure the woman has no preexisting blood-pressure condition, and to establish a baseline reading.

The baseline reading is the blood pressure that is normal for a particular patient; the doctor will check the blood pressure measurements at every other office visit against this baseline reading. In this way, the doctor can follow the pattern of change throughout the pregnancy.

The "pressure" in blood pressure refers to the force of the blood on the walls of your arteries. A blood-pressure reading, as you're probably aware, consists of two numbers, such as 120/80. The first number (the systolic pressure) shows the amount of pressure that's exerted against the walls of the artery during each beat of the heart. The second number (the diastolic pressure) is the pressure that's exerted *between* beats of the heart. Hypertension (high blood pressure) is defined as 140/90 or higher. If values this high are found in the first trimester, this would indicate chronic or preexisting hypertension, unrelated to pregnancy. Low blood-pressure values are much less worrisome, unless accompanied by symptoms such as lightheadedness and fainting.

During the second trimester, as the cardiovascular system changes to accommodate the growing pregnancy, blood pressure tends toward its lowest reading, then usually comes back up to baseline during the third trimester. At that point, blood pressures that rise above the base established at these first appointments can signal developing problems such as pregnancy-induced hypertension or preeclampsia (see page 137). Likewise, any reading that rises above 140 for systolic pressure or 90 for diastolic pressure will merit closer observation.

• **Urine sample.** As with blood pressure, the patient will give a urine sample at the first visit and then at every subsequent visit as well. The urine is tested with a reagent strip or "dipstick." The purpose of this test is to check for the presence of glucose or protein.

The presence of glucose, commonly known as sugar in the urine, might indicate the onset of gestational diabetes. Then again, it might simply indicate that the kidneys are filtering an increased amount of glucose, even though the blood levels are normal. Still, if glucose shows up repeatedly in a urine sample, the obstetrician will have to perform further tests to see if the patient is among the less than 4 percent of pregnant women who develop gestational diabetes (see page 144).

The presence of protein (also known as albumin) might indicate one of two potential problems:

1. *Bladder infection.* A further evaluation will determine whether this is indeed the case. Pregnant women are, unfortunately, at increased risk for bladder infections. (See "Urinary Tract Infections" later in this chapter.)

2. *Kidney dysfunction.* This can signal an underlying disease like lupus or the onset of preeclampsia. (See "Preeclampsia," page 137.)

If either of these is suspected, we'll retest a midstream urine sample with what we call a "long dip," which simply means a longer, more specialized test strip than the first test, or we'll send the urine out to a lab for more detailed testing.

• **Blood sample.** At the first visit, an obstetrician will take a complete blood count as well as perform routine blood tests to screen for hepatitis B, rubella immunity, and syphilis. If any of these results are abnormal, follow-up tests will be ordered. The doctor will also perform other tests, if relevant (such as a screen for toxoplasmosis, if a patient has a cat; see page 29), and every patient should also be offered a screen for HIV.

The doctor will find out your blood and Rh type, which determines if you have the potential for developing Rh incompatibility. When a woman is Rh negative, the baby's father should be tested as well. The results are known quickly—typically in a day. If you're found to be Rh positive, or you and your partner are both Rh negative, then there's no problem. But if you're Rh negative and your partner is Rh positive, then there can be incompatibility problems. In other words, if you and the fetus have different Rh factors, your body could read the baby's blood cells as foreign and reject them.

In that case, your body would generate a substance (also known as an antibody) that would attack the fetal red blood cells and cause the fetus to develop severe anemia. A woman who tests Rh negative, and whose partner does not, is therefore given injections of Rhogam, which protect her from producing antibodies: if any early bleeding occurs; at the time of an invasive procedure such as CVS or amniocentesis (see pages 38 and 105); again at 28 weeks; and then postpartum. Even if the pregnancy ends in miscarriage, Rhogam would be administered to a woman with Rh-negative blood, just in case she was exposed to fetal red blood cells.

PHYSICAL CHANGES

Not since the onset of adolescence has your body undergone such sudden, constant, significant changes. And no wonder. The same basic factor is at work: hormones, and lots of them.

Throughout this book, I'll cover the physical changes you can expect during each trimester of the pregnancy. In the first trimester, these include:

• **Breasts.** This is very likely the first significant area where you'll experience change, and it's a difference that can be especially dramatic among women who are usually small-chested. The breasts may grow in size and usually are tender for at least two to three months. The change in size is accompanied by a noticeable broadening and darkening of the areola (the area around the nipples), caused by an increase in the level of the melatonin-stimulating hormone affecting pigmentation; this will continue throughout pregnancy.

• **Vaginal secretions.** Also known as leukorrhea, this milky-white, watery vaginal discharge is often bothersome and embarrassing but a completely normal physiologic change. Many women find they have to wear a thin mini-pad throughout pregnancy.

• **Frequent need to urinate.** As the uterus expands, it increases pressure on the bladder, causing more frequent trips to the bathroom. This will diminish in the second trimester, as the uterus moves up and away from the bladder, but will return again—with a vengeance—in the third trimester, as the organs of the entire region feel the pressure of the head in the pelvis. Even if you find yourself constantly urinating, it's important that you continue to drink plenty of fluids.

• **Varicosities.** You'll probably notice new veins starting to pop up all over your body—in your breasts, along your abdomen, on the backs of your legs, and elsewhere (see "Vulvar varicosities" immediately below and "Hemorrhoids" on page 117). This is completely normal, and is the result of two changes in the blood distribution throughout your body: volume and drainage.

During pregnancy, your body has to produce more blood to accommodate the growing demands of the fetus. At the same time, the pressure of the expanding uterus on the veins compresses the blood flow. These two factors combine to weaken the protective valve system within the veins.

Your veins are designed to circulate the blood back to the heart, from all parts of the body. For obvious anatomical reasons, much of that journey is an exercise in antigravity, as the blood climbs back to the heart from (literally) the ground up, and that's where the protective valve system within the veins does its hardest work: The valves are supposed to prevent the blood from backing up in the veins. But because of the increase in blood volume and the compression of the return blood flow, the valve system gets an extra workout during pregnancy and soon weakens slightly. As it weakens, it allows for backflow, and the resulting pooling of blood shows up on the surface of your body as the bluish lines commonly called varicose veins.

While it's not, generally speaking, possible to totally *eliminate* varicosities during pregnancy, there are steps you can take to make the condition less pronounced:

1. *Don't stand or sit in one position for long periods.* If your job requires a great deal of standing, take care to sit down often and, if possible:

2. *Elevate your legs, which helps even out the blood flow in the areas of the body lower than the heart.*

3. *Wear support garments, including medical compression hose.*

Each pregnancy can add to the damage to the valve system, so varicosities will tend to manifest themselves earlier and more severely with each subsequent pregnancy.

Once the baby is born, and the blood volume drops and the pressure of the uterus on the veins relaxes, much, if not all, of the varicosities in the breasts and along the abdomen disappear.

• **Vulvar varicosities.** These first cousins to varicose veins are caused by increased blood flow, and result in the vaginal labia turning purple or blue and becoming distended. In some women, this can create a constant state of mild sexual arousal; in others, discomfort (see page 88). Vulvar varicosities almost always disappear soon after the baby is born.

• **Gums and nosebleeds.** You may feel very congested, a common side effect of the 40 percent increase in your body's total blood volume. Also, your gums may bleed easily, especially during brushing, and even during as benign an act as biting into an apple. Again, the increase in blood volume during pregnancy can cause the small capillaries to become full and traumatized. For this reason, good dental hygiene remains a priority during pregnancy.

Nosebleeds are common, too, because the blood vessels are so full. Recommended treatments include a saline solution for the nose and a humidifier in your bedroom.

FEELING BAD PHYSICALLY

You've probably heard other women speak about the struggle of the first trimester and the relative ease of the second. It doesn't always work on exactly this timetable, but know that if you're feeling lousy now it's a sign that everything is progressing as it should—that the hormones of pregnancy are hard at work on your entire body—and that, yes, the nausea *et cetera* will probably end by or around week 12 or 13. (For more on nausea, see page 56.) You may notice that the symptoms of pregnancy sometimes seem similar to the symptoms of menstruation—at least during a really, really bad period, the kind you used to get in high school.

Cramping in the first few weeks is *very common*, normal, and, as long as it's not accompanied by bleeding, nothing to worry about. (If it *is* accompanied by bleeding, see the "First-Trimester Bleeding" section later in this chapter on page 40.) Cramping is the reaction of the uterus to a fetus embedding itself in its muscular wall. As mentioned earlier, your breasts will be tender, too, and you might experience general fatigue, headaches, and achiness.

In short, during these early weeks you might just want to curl up in your bed for hours. All this will pass, and eventually the strange buzz of sensations and swellings will start to work in harmony to make you feel much better.

FEELING BAD EMOTIONALLY

Many people welcome the news of a pregnancy with joy, relief, unambivalent abandon. But many people don't, and the social pressure to do so can make a bad situation worse. I'm not talking about the occasional reservations, or the sudden, sinking, middle-of-the-night realization that from this day forward your life will never be the same. A pregnancy obviously comes with its own tremendous trunkful of emotional baggage, and a fair amount of hormonal carryons, too. Second thoughts are normal, maybe inevitable. The fact is, your life will *never* be the same again; why shouldn't you feel a little bit apprehensive?

The new hormonal flux of pregnancy can contribute to a pregnant woman's emotional highs and lows, but another matter entirely is true, diagnosable depression, the kind marked by dire and even dangerous thoughts. The twenties and thirties are, statistically, a prime age for depression in women to occur, whether they are pregnant or not. A seriously depressed pregnant woman will find herself not simply in a sensitive frame of mind—perhaps bursting into tears for no apparent reason—but unable to function. Sleeping, eating, concentrating, attending to details—the essentials of getting through daily life may seem beyond her. At its most extreme, the depression can grip its victim with thoughts of doing harm to herself and her unborn baby.

For many women, pregnancy is the happiest time of their lives. But for some, it's not, and if you suspect your unhappiness is excessive, you should tell your obstetrician immediately and seek psychological counseling, for your sake and the baby's.

ILLNESSES

Several illnesses have come to assume a special association with pregnancy—some because they're simply more common among pregnant women, and some because they pose possible threats to the health of the fetus. Within my experience, the following seem to be the illnesses that patients want to know about right from the start:

• **Chicken pox.** Ninety percent of adult women will have evidence of previous exposure to the chicken pox (varicella zoster) virus. These women (and their fetuses) are not at risk for developing the infection in pregnancy. Determining a patient's previous exposure often is simply a matter of asking her or her parents. If nobody's recollection is clear, and there is reason to believe that the woman has been exposed in pregnancy, then we can run a blood test to determine her immunity status. Sometimes the results of this test can be pleasantly surprising; a woman can find out that she's developed an immunity even if she doesn't remember having had chicken pox, if the case she had was mild enough.

If you think you might be among the 10 percent that aren't immune, however, then you'll want to take precautions. Chicken pox is highly contagious, and can be problematic, especially in the first half of the pregnancy. It can be transmitted transplacentally—from mother to fetus— and while the vast majority of women with chicken pox still deliver perfectly normal babies, the illness *can* lead to skin scars, intrauterine growth retardation, and abnormalities of the eye. If you are exposed to someone with chicken pox, you should know that once that person's lesions have crusted over, he or she is no longer contagious. If you have reason to believe that you've come in contact with someone who is suffering from chicken pox and is contagious, and you don't know your immunity status, contact your doctor immediately. (Be sure not to simply show up in the office with an undiagnosed rash that could be chicken pox, because you might put other pregnant women at risk.)

What, some of my patients have asked, would be the worst-case chicken pox scenario? A very dangerous time for a pregnant woman to *develop* chicken pox (and notice that I did not say "be exposed to"—they are two very different things) would be within the first twenty weeks, when congenital abnormalities can occur in the fetus. Because of the possibility of these abnormalities, an infected woman has to decide whether or not to continue her pregnancy. Also, if a woman were to develop active chicken pox very close to delivery, before she had a chance to develop immunity, her baby, when born, could become extremely sick (and so could she) and be at risk for life-threatening complications such as pneumonia. Treatment for the baby would include being injected with VZIG (varicella zoster immunoglobulin).

• **Rubella.** More commonly known as German measles, this is not usually a worry because of the universally administered (in the United States, at least) German measles vaccine. Immunity from vaccinations, however, can wane, and so even when patients insist that they've already had the shot, we'll still use the blood test at the first visit to determine their immunity status. (If a patient comes in for a pre-conception evaluation, we'll recommend that she be tested then; if she's found not to have the immunity, we'll vaccinate her and suggest she delay getting pregnant for 90 days.)

If a patient doesn't show immunity, we can't vaccinate her during pregnancy—but at least she'll know to take extra precautions. Exposure to rubella during pregnancy for a nonimmune woman, especially during the first trimester, can lead to serious birth defects, including central nervous system abnormalities. If a patient is nonimmune, fears she's been exposed (especially during the first trimester), gets tested for rubella, and tests show a very recent infection, she'll probably want to talk to her doctor and a genetics counselor about whether to proceed with the pregnancy.

• **Viruses.** Mild "bugs," both respiratory and intestinal, are a part of life, and pregnant women, unfortunately, aren't exempt from them. Most mild illnesses aren't a cause for serious concern, nor are the low-grade fevers that accompany them, which can be treated safely with extra fluids, bedrest, and Tylenol. (*Not* aspirin or ibuprofen-containing pain relievers such as Advil; for more on this restriction, see page 77. You should speak to your doctor, though, before taking *any* medication.) Any fever over 100.6 degrees Fahrenheit, while not necessarily dangerous to the fetus, should receive the immediate attention of your doctor, because it could be a sign of a bacterial infection, which might require antibiotics.

• **Urinary tract infections.** These are the most common complications of pregnancy, due to the physiologic changes in the urinary system at this time. In our practice (though not in all practices), we include a screen for asymptomatic (without symptoms) urinary infections at every visit. Pregnant women have an increased production of progesterone, a hormone that relaxes the smooth muscles and ligaments. There is also a decreased tone and incomplete emptying of the bladder, which can lead to an isolated bladder infection known as cystitis. The symptoms of this lower urinary tract infection include a frequent, urgent need to urinate, a burning sensation during urination, and, sometimes, abdominal pain. Treatment involves drinking plenty of fluids and taking antibiotics prescribed by your doctor.

As the smooth muscles that normally keep the urine moving between the kidney and the bladder begin to relax, the urine will "reflux" into the tube connecting the two and increase the chances for an upper urinary tract infection called pyelonephritis. This kidney infection, which can start out as cystitis, can cause high fever, chills, backache, and blood in the urine.

If you think you have a urinary tract infection, don't just rummage around in the medicine chest for any old antibiotics; you'll need a new prescription. Don't wait around to confirm your self-diagnosis; delay could cause worsening or progression to the more serious pyelonephritis. And if you think you have a kidney infection, you should pay a visit to your obstetrician immediately; you may even need to be hospitalized to receive intravenous antibiotics.

• **Toxoplasmosis.** This is a parasite infection that's most commonly acquired through contact with cat fecal matter, or by ingesting raw meat or touching utensils (or even another person's hands) that have had contact with raw meat. It can cause serious congenital abnormalities or even fetal death.

Don't be alarmed if your doctor suggests a test for toxoplasmosis and it comes back positive. These tests are done as early as possible in pregnancy—often they are included in the panel of tests done at the first visit. In 95 percent of these cases, the infection is not new and active, as a second test soon shows. It may indicate previous exposure only. But if the second test does show the infection to be new, then you should talk to your doctor about further testing.

I recommend several precautions:

1. *If you are a cat owner, minimize contact with kitty litter and the box.* A veterinarian could screen the cat to see if it's a carrier, but I'd still recommend precautions regardless of the test results.

2. *Never eat raw or undercooked meat, seafood, or eggs.*

3. *Observe strict hand-washing standards in the preparation of these foods.*

• **Lyme disease.** For every twenty women who call us worried that they've contracted Lyme disease, only one turns out to have it. The disease, which is classified as a type of arthritis, is found in the Mid-Atlantic states up through New England, the upper Midwest, and the far West. It is transmitted by a tiny tick called the deer tick, which lives in wooded areas.

Lyme disease sometimes shows up with a telltale, ring-shaped rash that grows larger in diameter over time, but often there is no rash. Other early symptoms include muscle aches and a low-grade fever. Left untreated, the disease can cause serious potential complications, including general arthritis and even organ damage. Potential fetal complications are less well understood; some studies have suggested the possibility of cardiac problems in the babies of some infected women. But there is no conclusive data, and we still don't know if there's a rational pattern to these cases, or whether they are random.

There are blood tests that can diagnose exposure to Lyme disease, and if a patient has been exposed she will be monitored over time and treated with antibiotics. I don't automatically treat every patient who has received a tick bite, but I do monitor them closely.

If you are going to be in a wooded area where deer ticks are found, you should take precautions. Stay out of long grass, wear pants, tuck your cuffs into the socks, and check yourself each evening for ticks or bites. If, despite these precautions, you are bitten by a deer tick, you shouldn't be hysterical, but should certainly discuss the situation with your doctor right away.

RISK OR FEAR OF MISCARRIAGE

Once I confirm the presence of a fetal heartbeat by sonogram—usually around the sixth or seventh week—I am relatively sanguine about the health of a pregnancy. (Again, if a sonogram isn't available to you at this stage, that's all right; it's helpful, but not an absolute medical necessity.) I wish I could say there is a zero risk of miscarriage at this point, but that's not so. The statistics are more like this: Before we find a heartbeat, the chance of miscarrying is close to 40 percent, believe it or not. (This includes the many, many women who never even know they were pregnant. Perhaps their period was late, and then the bleeding was particularly heavy. This might have been a miscarriage, and they never realized it.) After we find a heartbeat, though, the chance of miscarriage drops down to a 5 percent risk. (More on miscarriage under "First Trimester Bleeding" later in this chapter on page 40.)

This scenario is far different from what your mother or your friends might have been telling you: that the entire first trimester is a high-risk time. I still hear women who speak of their relief at reaching the 14th week, as though doctors, too, think of the end of the first trimester as a "whew" milestone in terms of not miscarrying. But in reality, we doctors are reassured at a much earlier point that you're probably not going to miscarry. When I pick up the presence of a heartbeat by ultrasound, or hear it with Doppler at eleven weeks, that, to me, is a cause for celebration. (The time between seeing and hearing the heartbeat, by the way, is usually about four or five weeks. We can now see an image of a pulsing heartbeat at six or seven weeks, as I mentioned. Our best Doppler machine—a device that sends out sound waves to detect motion—will pick it up at around 11 weeks, as opposed to 20 weeks in the not-too-distant old days.) Dopplers use much of the same technology as ultrasounds, but unlike ultrasounds they don't generate images from those sound waves.

As for when to tell people you're pregnant, that's a personal decision, based on your emotional makeup or ethnic superstition. (Though if you are in fact reluctant to tell people about your pregnancy even after a heartbeat has been found and your doctor says everything looks great, you may want to examine your feelings and fears.)

One particularly poignant reason some people wait to reveal a pregnancy is that they've had a previous miscarriage. I try to reassure them that the overwhelming majority of second pregnancies will not result in a repetition of what happened the previous time. Women do, as you know, sometimes experience two miscarriages in a row, but the cause of the first miscarriage may be very different from the cause of a second. Many women who experience one miscarriage will proceed more carefully through a subsequent pregnancy—sometimes even taking to bed—but this caution is not supported in medical literature. The fact is, the vast majority of early miscarriages are due to fetal genetic imperfections, and there's little you can do to alter their fate. Moreover, it used to be that we'd wait until a woman had experienced three first-trimester miscarriages before ordering further tests, but we now consider the odds against two consecutive first-trimester miscarriages to be long enough to merit a workup.

Most miscarriages occur very early and spontaneously in pregnancy. The later-in-gestation ones are much rarer, and in that case even one pregnancy loss in the second trimester would prompt us to consider whether the cause was an infection or a genetic abnormality or uterine anomaly. Although you probably know of some horrible story in which the friend of a friend lost a pregnancy quite late, you should know that it's rare to have a second-trimester miscarriage.

Second-trimester miscarriages are particularly traumatic because the woman has gotten attached to the fetus, has often felt movement, has made plans for the future. But first-trimester losses can be extremely traumatic, too. You worry that you'll never have a baby—that something is really *wrong* with you. Let me repeat that this is most likely not the case. Because, as I've mentioned, most early miscarriages are due to a fetal genetic imperfection, the loss of the pregnancy can be seen as a weeding-out of a fetus that wouldn't have thrived. These early miscarriages are a painful but real illustration of Darwin's theory of natural selection, which holds that what's physically superior survives, while what's not, doesn't.

GENETIC TESTING

Some of the more complex and occasionally controversial blood tests performed in the first trimester are genetic tests. These screening tests determine whether parents are *carriers* of a gene for a disease that could prove serious or even fatal to their children. Such testing can be done once pregnant, but ideally should be done pre-pregnancy, because what's being tested isn't the fetus but the parents—specifically, both parents are tested to see whether the combination of their genes may yield certain genetic diseases. A genetic counselor can then quantify the risk for a given disease in the offspring of that couple. When scheduling these tests during pregnancy, what's important to keep in mind is that it takes time to get the results and plan for testing of the fetus itself.

In most cases, both parents need to be carriers in order for their children to be affected. Such disorders are classified as "autosomal recessive," which means that if both parents are, in fact, carriers, then the child has a 25 percent chance of being affected. Some physicians will screen every woman at risk, and have her partner come in for testing if necessary.

There are a range of blood tests available to pregnant women and their partners; the decision to have them done is a personal choice. Most of the tests can either be performed by your doctor, or your doctor can refer you to a human genetics lab, where you and your partner can both be screened.

Bear in mind that genetics is a cutting-edge science, and that new tests are in the works that will eventually screen for a much wider range of disorders. But for now, here are the most common blood tests that patients and partners might elect to have done:

• **Cystic Fibrosis Screen.** This test screens for a disorder that affects the function of mucous and sweat glands, and is usually fatal in young adulthood. It appears more commonly among Caucasians than non-Caucasians. The likelihood of being a carrier is about 1 in 20.

• **Ashkenazic "triple-screen."** This panel is offered to patients of Ashkenazic Jewish descent, since the disorders it

screens for are more prevalent in this population. These disorders are all transmitted in an autosomal-recessive fashion,
requiring both parents to be carriers. Even if only one member of the couple is Ashkenazic, we still recommend that
both be screened; this decreases the chances of false-nega-
tive results. The panel includes Tay-Sachs (a fatal neurologic
disease), Gaucher, and Canavan diseases. Gaucher disease
is variable in nature. Infantile forms can be severe, with
neurologic involvement and shortened life span. Adult
forms can be mild, and may manifest themselves only in
enlargement of the spleen and liver, or in bone pain.
Canavan disease is a progressive neurologic disorder that is
fatal in early childhood. Since there is no known treatment
for Canavan disease, efforts are directed to prevention of the
disorder by carrier detection and prenatal diagnosis.

• **Sickle-cell anemia**, for African-American and Hispanic
couples. This is a hemoglobin disorder that causes severe
anemia which keeps oxygen from reaching body tissue and
organs. This leads to very painful crises and leaves patients
highly susceptible to serious infections. Sickle-cell anemia
is not curable and is often fatal in childhood or early adulthood. Again, both parents would have to be found to be carriers for the fetus to be at risk.

• **Thalassemia**, for couples of Mediterranean or Asian
descent. This is another anemia-type disorder that can lead
to liver damage, heart failure, and death in adolescence.
One strain of the disorder leads to a fatal disease called
Cooley's anemia.

Genetic testing in general, especially for some of the
rarer diseases, may not be something your doctor offers. In
fact, if your doctor doesn't routinely offer these tests, and
you tell him or her that you read about them in a book and

would like to have them done, he or she may look at you and say: *What in the world are you reading?*

The fact is that these tests are not considered "standard of care." They are, however, tests that I chose to have performed on myself when I was pregnant. If a patient is Caucasian, it's worth being tested for cystic fibrosis, because the carrier rate is about one in twenty. Even if only one member of a couple is Jewish I recommend the triple screen. African-American women should be screened for sickle cell trait since the carrier rate is 1 in 12. Women complain to me sometimes when I urge them to take the blood tests, saying: It's such a hassle, my husband doesn't want to miss work, blah, blah, blah.

I tell them this: *These diseases can be catastrophic.* Believe me, all it takes is contact with one heartbreaking family, in which the mother has delivered a Tay-Sachs baby, to make you want to screen the world.

And as for cystic fibrosis, if you're a Caucasian 35-year-old woman, you have a much greater chance of being a carrier of this disease than of having a Down syndrome baby.

Most books try to remain neutral on the topic of whether or not to test, and your own doctor may be neutral or even dismissive of your desire to have the screens performed. But as a doctor and a mother, I would urge you to seriously consider taking the relevant tests. We like to think that we're at a very advanced stage of medical research, in which we can ferret out all the potentially serious genetic problems a child can face, but in fact there are very few such problems we have the ability to test for. So my feeling is that the ones that we *can* test for, we should. Testing doesn't give you the answers about what to do, but it does give you information. If the information is available, don't you want it?

If you and your husband or partner were to be tested for Tay-Sachs, for instance, and found to be carriers, what would you do? Unlike the person who learns she has HIV and for whom drugs could change the HIV status of her baby, you can't alter the future health prospects for *your* baby. But you can enter into motherhood knowing that there's a 25 percent chance your child will be affected, and what that might mean. You might opt to undergo chorionic villus sampling or amniocentesis to ascertain fetal status. If you learn that your child will likely or definitely have a genetic disorder, you might opt to terminate the pregnancy. Or you might be more prepared by choosing a pediatric specialist in advance. You might even learn something that can be helpful for other family members; the results of a test might indicate that your other children and your siblings should be tested to determine if they carry certain genes, too. If you did receive a positive result on a test, your doctor would put you in touch with a genetics counselor, with whom you could discuss all of the possibilities, statistics, outcomes, and options.

Some patients have argued that these tests weren't done for thousands of years, so why should they be done now? It's true that life went on without genetic testing, and that millions of perfect babies were born to women who never had their blood drawn, but over those thousands of years, many terribly ill babies were also born.

I know, I know, I'm spooking you now. It's unpleasant to have to think about critically ill children at a time in your life when all you want to do is picture your newborn as perfect and healthy. I'm not trying to scare you unduly, only to share some of what I myself have witnessed as a doctor, and to tell you how it has affected my decisions as both a dispenser and receiver of medical care.

All tests, of course, have flaws. There are no "perfect" tests, and sometimes when I draw blood from a woman, I've unknowingly opened a genetic can of worms. You should know this before you decide to take any test. Some information is confusing and difficult to interpret; even the geneticists might not know what to make of a certain result. Will a positive result from a Gaucher's test mean that your child will be seriously ill? Or will it mean he might have almost no medical problems? No one can say for sure. But these are the kinds of questions that you and your partner and a genetics counselor can try to tackle, in the unlikely event that it becomes necessary.

I have a lot more to say on this topic with regard to other testing—sonograms, AFP screening, and, of course, the biggie, amniocentesis—but we'll deal with those questions when we get to the second-trimester section, as that's when those tests are made available.

CHORIONIC VILLUS SAMPLING

While I've been performing amniocentesis for years, in the recent past I've witnessed—and advocated—an increased usage of a procedure called CVS (chorionic villus sampling) in place of amnio. (For more on amnios, see p. 105.) Unlike the blood tests discussed above, CVS directly analyzes the genetic makeup of the fetus itself.

The main advantage of CVS over amnio is that it can be performed in the first trimester. So if the results are abnormal and you decide to terminate the pregnancy, the procedure is considered less difficult and less risky than in the second trimester. It's still a tremendous ordeal, of course, but of a somewhat different nature. The main disadvantage of CVS as opposed to amnio is that although it can be used to detect a great number of problems—a chromosomal abnormality such as Down syndrome, an enzyme deficiency such as Tay-Sachs, a gene defect such as sickle-cell anemia—it can't pick up anatomical anomalies such as open neural tube defects. (For more about neural tube defects, see page 101.)

CVS is performed by a specialist between weeks 10 to 12 (as opposed to 16 to 20 for an amniocentesis). This is how a CVS is performed: The woman lies on a table and a specialized catheter is inserted through her cervix and into her uterus. Most women say it doesn't hurt much at all. The doctor guides the path of the catheter by looking at an ultrasound monitor, and places the catheter between the lining of the uterus and the fetal membrane, which is called the chorion. The villi, which are fingerlike projections which form the placenta, can be cut off or suctioned out, and are taken to a lab to analyze. The villi offer a fairly thorough look at the chromosomes of the fetus.

Early statistics showed a significantly greater risk of miscarriage with CVS than with amniocentesis (one in 100 compared with one in 200), although my experience tells me both of those risk estimates are inflated. Both procedures have less risk when performed by experienced physicians. There have been limb abnormalities reported in babies whose mothers had CVS, but these situations seem to be directly related to the amount of experience of the person performing the procedure. Because CVS is still a fairly recently introduced procedure, you are well within your rights to find out how experienced this specialist is; a perinatologist usually has a referral practice and would have been doing these procedures on a regular basis.

In the past, I typically reserved my recommendations for CVS to women who were 40 or older, or whose babies were at increased risk for a specific genetic disorder, but my opinion is changing, and the age at which I might recommend it is getting lower. You should have a detailed discussion about this topic with your doctor, in order to decide what's best for you, based on your priorities and what makes you feel most comfortable.

First Trimester Bleeding

There are various hurdles throughout all three trimesters of a pregnancy, but as a doctor I don't view them as great challenges that a woman must meet—these aren't hurdles of a Herculean variety. Instead, I assume that a pregnancy will succeed unless I have specific reason to believe otherwise. After that very early miscarriage risk has passed, I feel more and more confident.

Bleeding is the biggest first-trimester concern. Many women experience some sort of bleeding, and if this happens you must always let your doctor know, describing the amount of blood and any cramping or pain. If you're bleeding and you've placed a call to your doctor and are waiting to hear back, you should lie down or sit in a comfortable chair with your feet elevated. Most likely your doctor will perform a sonogram, and maybe tell you to take it easy until the episode passes. Some episodes of bleeding do, of course, lead to miscarriage, but many more do not. If you have pain on one side, it could be caused by an ectopic pregnancy—although if you've already had an ultrasound, this condition would have been detected. Incidentally, another reason why an ultrasound is important is its ability to detect something called a molar pregnancy. The tissue inside the uterus does not form correctly, and can't progress normally. In the rare instance of a molar pregnancy, a woman would need a D&C (dilation and curettage) to empty the uterus.

If a miscarriage has already begun, then nothing can stop it. Sometimes a miscarriage occurs but isn't complete, and you will need to have a D&C to stop the bleeding. As I mentioned earlier, you may feel mournful about a miscarriage for a long time to come, and may be frightened to conceive again. But I can't tell you how many babies I've delivered to women who have had a previous miscarriage.

Bleeding doesn't necessarily mean that you are having a miscarriage. Your doctor will be able to tell by checking whether your cervix is dilated. If it's closed, and if an ultrasound shows that the fetus is still thriving, then you may very well be fine. (This situation is termed a "threatened abortion.") There are some women who simply bleed. It could be because of implantation bleeding; the fetus needs to make contact with the maternal blood supply—to invade, as it were, the mother's circulatory system in order to establish itself—and this can sometimes lead to bleeding. In a case like that, I would probably put the patient on pelvic rest (no sex, no tampons, no douching) until there's been no bleeding for seven days. Other possible causes of bleeding include an inflammation of the cervix, or a polyp that's dropped down into the canal due to the relaxation of the cervix.

I won't lie to you: As a doctor, I am concerned by bleeding, and I did worry that it would happen to me when I was pregnant. (It didn't.) If you start bleeding in a significant way, you will certainly get your doctor's attention. But you should know that we see bleeding in pregnancy all the time, and often it turns out to be a transitional occurrence that resolves on its own. As long as there's still a heartbeat, the pregnancy is stable.

Multiple Fetuses

Of course, there may be other *non*-routine concerns at this time, such as whether a patient is carrying twins. The number of twins (and triplets) in pregnancies is clearly on the rise as older women conceive and as more couples seek the aid of assisted reproductive technologies (such as ovulation induction and in vitro fertilization). The presence of more than one fetus will be definitively established at the first sonogram, but doctors will often have had their suspicions raised beforehand if uterine size seems greater than typical for the due date already established. Women carrying twins or triplets will be monitored over the months with extra sonograms—usually monthly—because it's otherwise difficult to assess how well the babies are growing. Generally, though, there's no reason that the pregnancy can't be a fairly routine one, and the pregnancy does not need to be followed by a high-risk specialist.

For the mother of multiples, the first trimester is not any different from that of a singleton except for the initial shock. Women carrying twins need extra folic acid; a supplement can be added to the prenatal vitamin she's already taking (for more on this, see p. 48). The amount of weight that mothers of twins gain can be extremely variable—anywhere from 30 to 50 pounds and upward—but the growth of each baby is the same as the growth of a singleton until about 32 weeks, after which a "crowding effect" begins.

Preexisting Medical Conditions

There may be some preexisting illnesses which require special attention during pregnancy. They include:

• **Chronic hypertension.** This refers to hypertension diagnosed either before the pregnancy or during the pregnancy but prior to the 20th week. By hypertension, we mean blood pressure readings over 140/90. It's important to determine whether women fall into this category because such readings indicate an increased risk for superimposed (meaning simultaneous) preeclampsia (see page 137) and *abruptio placenta*, the premature separation of the placenta from the uterine wall (for more on *abruptio placenta*, see page 84) and intrauterine growth restriction. As several of the medications that are frequently used to treat hypertension in non-pregnant women are not safe for use during pregnancy, these women are advised to seek prenatal care as early as possible so their medications can be adjusted or switched. Then during pregnancy, they're often followed more closely with special tests such as an electrocardiogram (EKG), echocardiogram (which is a sonogram of the heart), assessments of kidney function including 24-hour urine collection, serial ultrasounds (see page 97), and non-stress tests (page 138).

• **Asthma.** This is the most common obstructive pulmonary disease that coexists with pregnancy. The goals in following pregnant women with asthma are to decrease the number of attacks, to avoid severe attacks, and to maintain adequate oxygen supply. These women therefore should be encouraged to continue their asthma medications during pregnancy, including steroid inhalers, without fear of doing harm.

• **Seizure disorders.** If the patient hasn't experienced seizures in many years, we may try to wean her off her medications prior to pregnancy. Adequate control, however, is the most important aspect of therapy. If a patient needs to stay on anti-seizure medication, it's important to measure the levels of the medication in her blood throughout the pregnancy. It's also especially important for her to have a second-trimester anatomical ultrasound to rule out congenital anomalies associated with the use of certain anti-seizure medications. (For more on anatomical ultrasounds, see page 97.)

Whatever the circumstances of the individual patient, I'll want to make sure she's establishing healthy habits regarding nutrition (see the next chapter, page 47) and exercise (and the chapter after that, page 66). There may also be the aforementioned physical complaints such as nausea, breast tenderness, swelling, etc., that she'll want to address with me. But, truly, that's just about it. Sometimes I get the feeling the patient would prefer to hear that there are hundreds of contingencies on my mind. There are, of course, but a lot of the time our job—my job, and the patient's—is to get out of the way and let nature take its course. Trite, but true.

Although I'm a doctor, I'm not immune to the human element involved in a patient's pregnancy. We're not just talking medical events; we're talking families, entire lives being formed. While pregnancy is, again, not a disease, it *is* a time of intense bodily changes as well as intense concerns, anxieties, and fantasies, which will likely increase as these very weird and singular months go by.

Chapter Three
Table for Two

- •Diet
- •Morning Sickness
- •Cravings/Aversions
- •Weight Gain

Now, what about you?

At some point in the first two visits, after your doctor has finished reviewing the questions of greatest concern to her or him, you'll reciprocate: You'll ask the questions that are on *your* mind. If you're like most patients I know, you'll have been squirreling them away all week, lying awake in bed at three in the morning or waiting on line at the bank at three in the afternoon, saving them up for just this moment—the chance to produce what I've come to think of as "The List."

Of course, the medical issues I addressed in the last chapter involve you intimately—blood pressure, bleeding, even dating the pregnancy—but in all those cases, your participation is more or less passive. Those medical issues are the result of internal changes to your body, even when, like enlarged breasts, they manifest themselves externally. They're what happens to you because you're pregnant.

In this chapter and the next, I'll be addressing what happens to the pregnancy because of you. These are the areas where you take a more active role, where what you do can have a profound effect on the welfare of the fetus. It goes without saying that pregnancy is a big responsibility. So why am I saying it? Because the growing awareness of the nature of that responsibility is one of those experiences in life you can't really understand until you live through it. The first-trimester issues in these upcoming two chapters are all part of the slow but unmistakable strengthening of the bond—the inevitable recognition of the interdependence—between mother and child.

Which is where "The List" comes in. Some doctors freak out a little when patients pull out their endless lists, but I think they are great. A list is proof that the patient is taking her pregnancy seriously. A list often saves time later, when the patient is likely to telephone, saying, "There was something I forgot to ask you. . . ." And a list is especially useful for the patient, because pregnant women are notoriously forgetful. Whether this forgetfulness is due to hormones or distraction or anxiety no one is entirely sure, but a list will help you focus on everything that's been worrying you, and everything you're likely to worry about, no matter how absurd or trivial.

First rule: *Don't be shy.* Here's your chance to spill all. You'll want to be sure to ask about your doctor's recommendations on such matters as diet, exercise, travel, sex, testing, and, of course, delivery. Your first-trimester list should include all the burning issues you've thought of about matters both large and small. It can range from questions such as: What if my baby is retarded? to: What about stretch marks? I've had patients ask me if they can dent the baby's head by pushing on the belly (for the record: no) or if they can tell the baby's sex by looking in the mirror at their own faces (ditto).

If you do forget to ask something during the office visit, just remember: That's what phones are for. I always tell my patients to call with questions, though if it's not an emergency, to save it for office hours. (I say this with a chuckle, but I'm dead serious. I've actually been awakened at 3:00 A.M. by a woman wanting to know if it was okay that she ate half a dozen Godiva chocolates that day. And don't even *think* about calling me while *Melrose Place* is on!)

DIET

This section of the book is going to be a lot shorter than you might have expected. Still, it's a topic of such complexity and widespread interest that it (and its related issues) deserves a chapter all its own.

Women in our culture have all kinds of problems with body image, as you no doubt already know, and sometimes pregnancy only serves to emphasize these problems. As far as the whole matter of diet goes, I tend to take a very laid-back approach. I am a doctor, but when I was pregnant, did I sit there counting calories and protein intake, weighing foods and making sure I was getting the appropriate amounts of everything my body and my little brine shrimp–sized fetuses needed?

The answer is, emphatically, no.

I did not obsess over these questions, because I understood, as a doctor, that it wasn't necessary. Some pregnancy

books try to scare you into counting out the fat grams, calories, and God knows what else of everything you eat. Some
books try to give you an additional guilt trip about eating
sweets. I don't think that's necessary. Many foods in the
American diet are enriched, and, to quote the wisdom of
grandmothers: *The baby takes what it needs.*

This is a mantra that you should remember when you
wake up at 3:00 A.M. in a panicky state, convinced that you
didn't eat enough protein that day. The baby does take what
it needs. The "baby," who, right now, more closely resembles a fava bean than it does either you or your husband, is
most likely getting everything it needs if, prior to being
pregnant, you followed a reasonable diet.

Once again, *pregnancy is not a disease.* As with many
other areas of pregnancy, if you take a common-sense
approach to diet, you'll be much better off than polling
family, friends, and strangers on every last question. Boil
down everything we know about nutrition and pregnancy,
and there aren't that many significant changes a pregnant
woman needs to make.

Having said that, I would be remiss if I didn't emphasize
that a few new demands do require special attention:

• **Prenatal vitamins.** Those horse-pill prenatal vitamins,
which virtually every doctor will prescribe, can be intimidat-
ing, and many patients ask if such supplements are really
necessary in today's "multi-" and "-enriched" era. Probably
not. But I still want my patients to take them. I'm fairly confident that my patients are being adequately nourished, and
that their babies are reaping the benefits. But these vitamins are specifically designed for pregnant women; the
doses of the different vitamins and minerals have been
carefully calibrated.

Ideally, a patient would have been taking a prenatal vitamin prior to getting pregnant. Because half the pregnancies in the United States are unplanned, medical groups now advise *all* women of childbearing age to take prenatal vitamins, especially for their folic acid component. Studies have conclusively shown that neural tube defects can be prevented by folic acid supplementation, and the prenatal vitamins include enough folic acid to help prevent these defects, which occur fairly soon after conception. But if you haven't taken them, there's no cause for alarm; the incidence of neural tube defects in the general population is only 1 in 1,000 births.

Aside from the neural tube concern, the use of prenatal vitamins is somewhat of a reflex on the part of the medical establishment and mothers-to-be. Just as it makes sense for the part of the population that isn't pregnant to take multivitamins, it makes sense for pregnant women to take those vitamins that are specially designed for their use. Ideally, if a woman were to follow the "letter of the law" regarding nutrition (see following sections), she would have no need for additional nutrients. But it's virtually impossible to follow an absolutely ideal diet—so why not supplement?

By the way, don't ever substitute "regular" vitamins for prenatal vitamins. What counts as a regular vitamin these days—including pills that advertise themselves as megavitamins, and that contain absurdly high amounts of things you don't really need absurdly high amounts of—can be harmful to pregnant women. (Sometimes, for example, they're chock-full of vitamin A, which, in massive doses, has been linked to birth defects of the central nervous system and elsewhere.)

If you can't tolerate the prenatal vitamins (some women

are nauseated by them), I'd rather that you take a break from them for a week or two, then try again. And then, if you really can't hold them down, you might switch to a children's chewable vitamin and a folic acid supplement, which at least will give you some of what you need without too much bother. I know, you may feel a bit ridiculous chomping on Wilma Flintstone, but I think it's a good idea. Once the nausea passes, you can try the prenatal vitamins again.

• **Calcium.** Calcium intake is crucial because it contributes to the development of the baby's teeth, bones, muscles, nerves, and heart, among other body parts. It also replaces the calcium that's being drawn out of your bones to supply the fetus, and reduces your risk for osteoporosis.

You'll need four 8-ounce servings a day of milk—or the equivalent in other calcium-rich foods. Each 8-ounce serving of milk carries about 300 mg. of calcium, so if you're devising your own calcium-intake diet you'll need to come up with approximately 1,200 mg. of calcium. Here are some common dairy equivalencies, showing milligrams of calcium per serving:

Hard cheese:	1 oz. American cheese, 195 mg.
	1 oz. Swiss cheese, 259 mg.
Soft cheese:	1 oz. cream cheese, 23 mg.
Yogurt:	8 oz. low-fat, 275 mg.

By the way, skim milk is recommended rather than whole milk (or whole-milk products) because it will provide calcium without the additional unnecessary calories. These days, calcium-rich orange juice exists, and each glass of it provides as much calcium as a glass of milk.

Two other common calcium-rich substitutes are canned salmon (with bones), a 3.5 oz. serving of which yields 200 mg. of calcium, and tofu processed with calcium, a 3.5 oz. serving of which yields 128 mg. Peas, broccoli, and dark green leafy vegetables (except spinach) will also provide some calcium; 2/3 cup of cooked broccoli, for instance, yields 88 mg., and 1/2 cup of cooked collard greens yields 150 mg. And while I can't vouch for it myself, the medical guide I've got here on my desk says that a 3 oz. serving of either raw seaweed or kelp will give you a whopping 1,000 mg. of calcium—virtually your entire daily requirement.

And then there are Tums and Rolaids, which also contain calcium. When women ask me whether they can skip milk entirely and just get everything they need from Tums or over-the-counter supplements, I tell them no (with some exceptions, such as for lactose-intolerant patients). Dietary sources are far better; they give you the vitamin D you need, as well as the calories. Tums or Rolaids, if taken to excess for their calcium content, can give you too much of what of you *don't* need. In any event, never take more than what the label directs. Women who ask about this substitution are usually searching for the easy fix: the pill they can take instead of drinking milk or eating cheese. Better to take a deep breath and drink the milk itself.

• **Fluids.** You'll need about eight glasses of fluid a day, and this can include your calcium needs. For instance, you can have three to four glasses of skim milk, plus four more of whatever (nonalcoholic) beverage you like.

• **Iron.** As mentioned in the previous chapter, during pregnancy, your body experiences a 25 percent increase in the production of red blood cells, just to meet your higher metabolic demands. For that reason, you'll need to supplement your iron intake. Some good sources of iron are red meat, especially liver; enriched breads and grains; and raisins.

By the way, studies indicate that your body absorbs iron better when Vitamin C is consumed at the same meal, so you can drink a glass of orange juice with a vitamin pill and meet several of your dietary needs in one sitting (fluid, iron, and, if it's the right kind of o.j., calcium).

• **Folic acid.** As mentioned earlier, folic acid helps prevent neural tube defects. Good sources include leafy green vegetables, liver, fruits, and cereals fortified with folic acid.

• **Extra calories.** Basically, you'll need to consume roughly 300 more calories a day than you did before you were pregnant, but I don't think you need to fret over this, or to waste time counting calories. You will be able to bulk up your diet without even trying, because you'll find yourself increasingly hungry.

• **Fiber.** In addition to fluids and exercise, increasing your fiber intake can alleviate constipation. Good sources of fiber include bran cereal, prunes, raisins, and almonds. Fresh fruits and vegetables with seeds or skin contain more fiber.

• **A well-balanced diet.** There really isn't much more to say than what my fifth-grade teacher used to say when she whipped out her "Basic 4" food chart: Try to eat protein, dairy, grains, fruits and vegetables every day. If you follow your common sense, you'll know not to sit there eating Marshmallow Fluff from a jar. (At least, not all the time.) Obviously, if you're choosing between an apple and a Milky Way, the apple is healthier, just as it is when you're not pregnant—and as you have two mouths to feed, why not go for the healthy choice? But it's no crime to cave in to a craving. Eat what you enjoy, and be sure to include those things your teacher told you about. The American diet has become so varied that "grains" can mean risotto, cooked with plenty of calcium-rich cheese. You can even throw a little nouvelle cuisine into the mix. By and large, you can simply do what's sensible. You already know what to eat, without even knowing that you know. Green leafy vegetables, fruits, cheeses, good sources of protein such as beans or red meat . . . need I go on? You should eat heartily, and frequently, and healthily, and if the scale shows you're gaining weight, then you're probably doing fine.

But just in case you're really worried that you're going to undernourish your fetus, I've included a sample one-day diet for a pregnant woman, to give you an indication of the way you should be eating (and the way you probably already are):

Breakfast:	2 slices whole wheat bread
	1 tbs. peanut butter
	1/2 cantaloupe
	1 cup skim milk
A.M. snack:	1 cup yogurt
	1 banana
Lunch:	turkey sandwich on rye bread
	lettuce and tomato
	soft drink
	1 apple
P.M. snack:	2 Fig Newtons
	1 cup skim milk
Dinner:	1/2 roasted chicken
	green salad with 2 tbs. dressing
	sweet potato with 1 tsp. margarine
	1 cup skim milk

Late snack:	2 scoops ice cream	
Summary for day:	calories	2200
	carbohydrates	55%
	fat	25%
	protein	20%
	fiber	30 grams
	calcium	1500 mg.

You can see from this menu that while it satisfies essential nutritional needs, it's not terribly austere. I've included a soft drink, which is entirely optional and serves no function other than to make life slightly more pleasurable. Also note the presence of certain calcium-rich foods such as yogurt and ice cream. Leafy green vegetables contain calcium and essential vitamins and minerals, so try to include these when planning meals. If you're eating out in a restaurant and ordering an entree, it helps to pay attention to details. What side dishes, if any, does the meal come with? Supplement meat or fish with a grain and a vegetable.

• **Restrictions.** As you probably know, raw or undercooked chicken or eggs can house salmonella and other bacteria. The best safeguard, I think, is to order everything done medium-well, and to save the sushi for your first-night-at-home-with-the-baby take-out dinner. With regard to ground beef, due to the spread of the dangerous bacterium *E. coli* in recent years, you ought to cook hamburgers and meat loaf extra thoroughly—which means until there's no pink left inside.

Some patients worry about eating *any* sort of fish because of reports of elevated mercury levels, but I tell them that studies of populations whose diets consist mainly of freshwater fish show no evidence of adverse neurologic outcomes.

Also beware of unpasteurized dairy products, which might harbor the dangerous listeria bacterium. When buying cheese, always make sure it's pasteurized.

Some of the more exotic herbal teas supposedly can cause complications and even induce labor. I've never knowingly encountered any such occurrences, but if you come across a strange brew of any sort (outside the garden-variety Celestial Seasonings–type kind of assortment), it certainly couldn't hurt to consult with your doctor before imbibing.

MORNING SICKNESS

The consumption of milk, cheese, iron supplements, or anything else can seem entirely beside the point, if you're one of the many women who experience pregnancy-related nausea. This is something that, if it occurs, is bound to change your entire approach to food. The idea of having to eat or drink *anything* when you don't feel like eating at all, but in fact feel like curling up like an old dog and perhaps dying, may seem absurd. You may worry that when you can't eat you're depriving your baby, and that he or she will suffer because of it. I can say with great medical certainty that this isn't true. Again, as with most other considerations concerning diet, nature isn't always quite as exacting as you might think.

First, we should distinguish between three forms of gastrointestinal distress that occur during pregnancy. In ascending order of severity, they are: esophageal reflux, nausea and occasional vomiting, and hyperemesis, which is *extreme* nausea and vomiting. Strictly speaking, only the less extreme version of nausea and vomiting is generally considered morning sickness, but as all three share symptoms, women often have trouble telling them apart. For your own peace of mind, and even for health reasons that will soon become apparent, I recommend you make the effort to figure out which (if any) applies to you:

• **Esophageal reflux (heartburn).** As I mentioned in the last chapter, a hormone called progesterone relaxes the smooth muscles in a pregnant woman. Progesterone relaxes the lower esophageal sphincter, a theoretically one-way valve separating the esophagus from the stomach. As a result, food and acidic gastric juices backflow from the stomach into the esophagus, creating a burning sensation in the center of the chest. As the pregnancy progresses, this discomfort is compounded by a slowing of the digestive process—a development which helps your body absorb the nutrients the fetus needs, but which doesn't help your heartburn. As a result, reflux, which can strike as early as the first trimester, usually only gets worse as the pregnancy stretches on and on.

Almost every pregnant woman will suffer her share of gastrointestinal indignities, but you can help alleviate the burning sensation that accompanies reflux through taking antacids such as Tums, eating smaller but more frequent meals, and maintaining a non-horizontal posture for three hours after meals.

• **Nausea and occasional vomiting.** Morning sickness is a misnomer. It can strike any time of day (or all the time), and it can cause significant distress. Generally it hits in the first trimester and resolves by a magical twelve- or thirteen-week mark.

Having said that, I must admit that I was one of the lucky ones who for some reason got off scot-free. I was apprehensive when I found out I was pregnant with twins; some theories assert that because the hormone levels are so high, morning sickness in multiple births can be even worse. So I braced myself, preparing for a tidal wave. What can I say? It never came. There's probably a genetic component at work here; my mother tolerated early pregnancy well. You might want to ask your own mother what she experienced, for this could provide a somewhat reliable predictor of what your experience will be.

Unfortunately, we don't understand nausea. We don't know why the body sometimes seems to rebel early in pregnancy. When doctors don't understand what causes a problem, it's difficult to treat it. But I have collected various pieces of homespun wisdom from my patients as to what works for them, from which I have compiled the following catalog of remedies, all of which have helped some of my patients to one degree or another:

1. *Eat more frequently but in smaller quantities.*

2. *Take your prenatal vitamins at night rather than in the morning.*

3. *Take liquid antacids,* which seem to be more effective than tablet forms.

4. *Try seabands or acupressure bands.*

5. *Consider the use of pharmacological medications, some over the counter (Benadryl, Unisom), some prescription.* But *never* take them without first asking your doctor.

6. *Keep food in the stomach.* Crackers by the bedside, for instance, can provide a perfect pick-me-up (and keep-it-down).

• **Extreme nausea and vomiting.** A word of caution is in order here. Some women experience an extreme form of nausea and vomiting, also known as hyperemesis, that borders on unendurable, and try to tough it out because they figure that's what pregnant women do. The confusion between morning sickness and the more debilitating, and potentially dangerous, hyperemesis is compounded by the fact that both peak in the first trimester. Typically, the majority of symptoms associated with both morning sickness and hyperemesis abates by the second trimester. That's not to say that there won't be a bad day here and there, but most women feel significantly better by week 13.

When a woman calls and complains about her morning sickness, I'll assume the fact that she's calling is itself a sign of how serious the situation is, and I'll want to know two things: Is she vomiting excessively? Is she incapable of keeping liquids down? If the answer to either question is yes, I'll order tests on the electrolyte status of her blood and the concentration of her urine to see if her liquid intake is keeping up with the body's needs. If it turns out she's in danger of dehydration, I'll either hospitalize her or, as is increasingly common these days, put her on home intravenous hydration.

Also, it's always possible that what seems like hyperemesis could in fact be a gastrointestinal bug or a gallbladder problem. If you have any doubt—if what you're suffering seems as if it might be well beyond the normal—don't hesitate to call your obstetrician (a good rule to keep in mind for any aspect of pregnancy).

CRAVINGS AND AVERSIONS

Some women have cravings, and have them bad. I've had women in my office who crave red meat so badly, they're practically like cavemen in their voraciousness. Cravings, like morning sickness, are not really understood by doctors. One theory to explain cravings, as you've probably heard, holds that a body lacking certain minerals or iron tries to make up for these deficits. (Maybe that's why you never seem to hear about cravings for sweets—strong fondnesses, maybe, but not intense cravings; it's almost as though we're biologically programmed not to crave these foods because they're not useful to us from a nutritional point of view.) In extreme situations, women develop pica, in which they crave and even eat inappropriate substances such as cornstarch, mud, chalk, or laundry detergent.

After hearing wild stories from pregnant patients—like the woman who would scrape ice out of the bottom of the freezer because she enjoyed the metallic taste—I kept waiting for wicked cravings to hit. I was prepared to act out an episode of "I Love Lucy," in which I would make my husband, Jeff, run out in the middle of the night like Ricky Ricardo to fetch me sour pickles and ice cream. In fact, my actual experience was quite different. While I had no cravings for particular foods, I did become wildly hungry at times, in such a way that I needed to eat *then and there*. And if I didn't, I felt as though I would pass out. As both a doctor and former near-fainter-from-hunger, I would advise you to keep food in your bag or briefcase or whatever it is you carry with you during the day. Crackers, cookies, fruit, juice, pretzels, rice cakes, bagel chips, dry cereal, even—*gasp!*—something decadent and filled with empty calories like a Snickers bar will do the trick. There might well be moments when you feel a low-blood-sugar lightheadedness, a hollowness in your stomach, and a panicky need to eat. (This is especially true during the first trimester, when you'll probably notice the most significant changes in appetite.) Have something readily available—a quick fix—and you'll feel better.

The opposite phenomenon—aversions—also occurs frequently. As with cravings, we don't really understand what causes aversions, either. Smells often trigger these feelings of disgust, and for some reason Chinese food seems to top the list. So the first months of your pregnancy may not be spent in a euphoria of take-out Double Happiness Chicken, as you had planned. But take heart: In the same way that cravings might be the body's way of forcing you to get what you need, maybe aversions are the body's way of keeping you away from what you don't.

Whatever your present circumstances—craving, aversion, or steady-as-she-goes—I can tell you with reasonable certainty that if you ate fairly well before you were pregnant, and you're trying your best to eat well now, you are doing just fine.

WEIGHT GAIN

If you started your pregnancy weighing roughly what you ideally should be weighing for your height, I'd like to see you gain between 25 and 35 pounds. Here are a couple of quick rules of thumb that doctors use when thinking about a patient's weight:

• **Ideal pre-pregnancy weight.** Start with a height of five feet and a weight of 100 pounds, and for every inch over that add five or six pounds. That's your ideal weight (adjusted, of course, for your particular body frame).

• **Ideal weight gain during pregnancy.** This follows a simple trimester-by-trimester, 5-, 15-, 10-pound-gain formula. In the second and third trimesters, you can also think of this as *roughly* one pound per week.

If you started your pregnancy overweight, this certainly is not the time to try to lose weight. You may feel a bit worried about gaining more weight now, but you're going to have to put aside your vanity and your fantasies once and for all about losing your extra pounds. Remember, pregnancy lasts only nine months, and eventually the baby will be born and then you will have another chance to face the dreaded issue of weight loss. (Though there are some weight-loss programs for overweight pregnant women. Ask your doctor.)

If you're obese, however, you shouldn't gain too much — probably between 15 and 20 pounds. There are several obvious reasons for this recommendation: impaired mobility, general discomfort, weakening of the joints. There are also a couple of less obvious but well-known reasons: Obesity can put pregnant women at risk for diabetes (see page 144) and hypertension (page 137). But there's another, even more subtle medical reason for having overweight women gain less weight than average-weighted women: They have a tendency to deliver macrosomic babies—those weighing 4,000 grams (over 8 pounds, 13 ounces.)

Macrosomic babies tend to have a different distribution of their body fat from most babies. Usually the largest part of an average baby's body is the head, and once it passes through the birth canal we're all home free—mother, newborn, and obstetrician. But a macrosomic baby's weight is distributed so that the part of the body below the neck is disproportionately large. One of the most frightening situations that an obstetrician can encounter in the labor room (and one that happens in a reported one out of 300 live births) is when the head is delivered and then gets sucked back in, a situation known as the "turtle sign." This is often a harbinger of something called shoulder dystocia, in which the shoulders literally get stuck mid-delivery, and which can lead to a palsy in the baby's arm and other serious complications. So, to avoid such a potentially scary situation, we try to keep babies from becoming macrosomic in the first place.

Any of these dietary recommendations, of course, is subject to revision if a patient has special needs—if, for instance, she is a vegetarian, or has a lactose intolerance, or has a history of an eating disorder. If you're a vegetarian, you'll need to discuss alternative ways of getting protein (but probably you already know what these are). Lactose intolerance is less of a difficult issue these days thanks to lactose-reduced and lactose-free dairy products, which are widely available, and which provide the same amount of calcium as their lactose-loaded relatives.

Bulimic and anorexic patients generally don't deal well with getting on the scale at visits. The weighing-in is as much a part of a pregnancy visit as it is of a Weight Watchers meeting, yet for a woman with a severe eating disorder I'm willing to make a special exception and allow her to skip the weighing-in; it may be extremely difficult for her to face the numbers on a scale, and I don't want to torment a patient. I have other ways of seeing if the fetus is thriving. I can get a sense just by looking at a patient, asking about her diet, and by feeling her abdomen to check the fundal height (uterine size), which lets me see whether the uterus is expanding upward as it should be.

If you have an eating disorder and are truly troubled by the scale, ask your doctor if you might forgo this part of the routine. In that case, it will be essential for you to have supervision to help you nourish the fetus. Yes, the baby takes what it needs, but you have to be able to give it something from which to take, and to do so you'll probably need the assistance of a nutritionist. It will be helpful for you to have someone to talk to during pregnancy, and it will be helpful for your obstetrician to have someone to talk to about your particular needs, if necessary.

There are some women who gain considerably more than is recommended. When this happens, the first thing to consider is whether there's a genetic component at work. I ask these women to find out among the women in their families who have children whether they too gained an excessive amount of weight when they were pregnant. If this turns out to be the case, then controlling the weight gain may simply be impossible for these patients. I make sure they don't feel guilty or bad about themselves, and I reassure them about their ability to return to their normal weight after the pregnancy is over. Also, they may want to focus on being sure to return to pre-pregnancy weight before the next pregnancy.

For most women—ones of average weight who don't have eating disorders—the idea of eating liberally, and with gusto, with the aim of gaining weight, can be both liberating and a bit daunting. We've been instructed along far different lines pretty much since adolescence, and now it's time to chuck many of our long-held notions and eat for two. Back in our mothers' day, women were advised not to gain much weight, and I heard of one woman who, in the early 1960s, gained something like seven pounds and paraded her slimness with pride. But we now know that, for optimal results, you need to gain much more than that. So when you're feeling up to it (which, for women who bypass morning sickness entirely, may be right away), you should take pleasure in what you eat.

Chapter Four

No Regrets

- Exercise
- Stress
- Travel
- Caffeine
- Smoking
- Alcohol and Drugs
- Sexually Transmitted Diseases
- Sex

What have I done wrong?

Almost every patient I've ever seen has asked me some variation on that question at some point during the first couple of appointments. Usually the question doesn't take quite so direct or self-critical a form, but it's there, all right: the fear that some minor (or not-so-minor) indulgence, some little lapse in judgment—or even some ongoing everyday activity that, outside the boundaries of a pregnancy, might be laudable, such as exercise—has somehow harmed the baby.

We're so used to thinking only of ourselves when it

comes to what we eat or drink or how we behave, that at first it might be difficult to remember that being pregnant means there's actually someone else in there, someone who can be affected by our actions. And then it becomes just as difficult not to regard the memory of each transgression as if it were going to turn into a "Eureka!" moment some months down the line—the reason, in retrospect, why something's gone wrong.

First, let me assure you that it's difficult to harm a fetus, as nature has ways of shielding the next of kin from any number of ill-advised ventures on the part of the mother. I'm not saying that it's *impossible* to harm a fetus; there are, of course, certain activities a pregnant woman absolutely should avoid. And yet, chances are, should a complication arise, nothing the mother did—no drug she took, no cigarette she inhaled, no glass of Chablis she drank—is the cause, and the added pain of guilt and finger-pointing won't help anyone, least of all the baby.

So let's address these concerns calmly and slowly, one at a time.

EXERCISE

Patients come to me and ask exactly—and I mean *exactly*—what is safe to include in their pregnancy regimen. Is it okay to lift ten pounds of weight at the gym? How about eleven? They look at me intently, waiting for answers, and I know that what I say matters to them deeply; these tend to be women for whom the gym is very important. They've been taking good care of their bodies for years, and it shows. I have to sigh inwardly during these conversations, because "correct" amounts of exercise are very difficult to establish. I can't dictate exactly how much weight these women should lift, or how many repetitions are safe. Still, I can offer a few general rules of thumb:

• **Thirty to sixty minutes, three or four times a week.** If you're looking for a specific formula on how much or often to exercise, there it is. (But, as with most formulas for pregnant women, you still have to use common sense. If you're the kind of exercise enthusiast who thinks she can continue to do it all . . . well, you can't. You still have to listen to what your body is saying—now more than ever.)

• **Swim.** Likewise, if you're looking for a specific exercise, this is it. Swimming is perfect for pregnant women. It's not weight-bearing, it's a good aerobic exercise without stress, and it keeps you cool.

• **Avoid excessive heat.** Saunas, Jacuzzis, hot baths—all extremes of temperature should be avoided, though bathing is no problem, nor swimming in warm water. In the first trimester, the embryo is at a critical stage of development, and high temperatures can cause maldevelopment. Sweating is our mechanism of controlling the level of body heat, and you have to remember that, unlike us, a fetus can't cool down by sweating. We cool down by getting our water to evaporate into the air, while a fetus is surrounded by nothing *but* water. The body heat of the fetus has literally nowhere to go. Also, the body is already working hard enough at rest; when it heats up, the body has to work even harder to cool down. So the principle to remember in general is to avoid anything that elevates the core body temperature, which, of course, is 98.6—in a word, warm, not *hot*.

• **Make sure that you are able to carry on a conversation.** No matter what form your exercise takes or how long it lasts, imposing this one condition on yourself is an easy way to limit the level of strenuousness.

- **Keep your heart rate under 140.** Over that limit, your blood flow will be shunted toward your own skeleto-muscular structure, at the expense of the uterus and fetus.
- **Keep well-hydrated.**
- **Always exercise in a well-ventilated area.**
- **Don't change—***modify.* If you were physically active before you got pregnant, you can keep being physically active now—but bear in mind that your joints have become lax due to the increasing production of the hormone relaxin, which has the effect of relaxing ligaments throughout your body. This relaxation of the joints is only going to continue; it will even accelerate in the third trimester. In pacing your exercise regimen as the pregnancy progresses, you therefore must keep in mind that you'll be more and more prone to injury.

Some pregnant women swear by the formula of taking down the level of the workout by one-third or one-half; this is fine as far as it goes, but again, I prefer not to be so specific. Such thinking almost inevitably prompts a few people to regard a simple quantification as if it were a commandment, even as it violates what their own aches and exhaustion (to say nothing of common sense) are telling them. You'd be better off, I think, to try to shift your exercise program to include less of the kind of activity which entails frequent side-to-side movement or bouncing around on your knees and ankles. Think "low impact." The treadmill and Stairmaster are good, and so is the stationary bike, although your expanding body might get uncomfortable on that tiny seat. The new recumbent cycles seem popular. In general, I like the staying-in-place forms of exercise because, as your center of gravity shifts, you'll become more unstable than you might think.

(The American College of Obstetricians and Gynecologists has endorsed a videotape called "The Pregnancy Exercise Program," which is available from Health Point at 1-800-697-9987.)

If you work out at a gym with a trainer, be sure to let him or her know that you're pregnant, in case specific modifications need to be made. Avoid the kind of floor exercises that keep you on your back for long periods. Abdominals can be done through 20 weeks or so, as long as you're not performing them on your back for an extended time. (You can also do them on your side, by the way.) The main thing is: *As soon as any exercise becomes uncomfortable, that's the signal to stop.*

Some forms of exercise that sound great for pregnant women, such as yoga, are not especially wise to take up at this point as a beginner. They easily can prove to be more strenuous than you think, stretching new back and stomach muscles.

By the same token, if you're sedentary to begin with, pregnancy is not the time to *start* a strenuous regimen. You can try the low-impact exercises recommended above—the treadmill, Stairmaster, stationary bike—as long as they don't hurt you or cause fatigue. Not surprisingly, studies show that pregnant women who exercise feel better, both mentally *and* physically. Most exercise helps in particular with one of the most common pregnancy and post-pregnancy complaints, the dreaded lower back pain.

And now, a minority opinion: I know that many women swear by Kegel exercises, and there are prenatal classes that stress their use. The principle behind the Kegel is that by repeatedly tightening your vaginal and anal muscles you can strengthen your perineum, thereby reducing the chances of needing an episiotomy. Personally, I doubt it. In fact, a well-toned perineum might not have as much "give" at the time of delivery; in other words, it might actually *increase* your chances of needing an episiotomy. My advice: Don't bother.

(Post-delivery Kegel exercises, however, can help decrease or eliminate incontinence, which is linked to a weakening of the perineum due to the stress on the pelvic floor during pregnancy and to the pushing during delivery—but that's another story.)

As for my own pregnancy, I must shamefully admit that my exercise regimen was nearly nonexistent, falling under the heading of "sedentary." Except for taking some brisk walks around the Central Park Reservoir and delivering babies, I didn't do much in the way of physical activity. Which doesn't mean that you should follow my lead; in fact, I hope you don't.

• **Use common sense.** This is a blanket statement that covers any number of subjects in this book, but it's one well worth repeating here. Now is not the time in your life to "make it burn." If it hurts, stop. Likewise, if it's potentially harmful to the fetus, *don't do it.*

This is especially true when you leave the confines of your exercise mat or gym for more rugged terrain. Patients ask if they can downhill ski when they're on vacation. Yes, they'll probably be just fine, but some sort of accident could happen, and do you really want to put your baby in jeopardy for the sake of a totally unnecessary activity? The same is true for riding a bicycle, even if your pedaling skill is practically up to *Breaking Away* standards. Remember: Your center of gravity has shifted, and everything is slightly *off*. I had a patient in her seventh month who asked me if she could go snowmobiling when she was on vacation, and I just gave her an "Are you for real?" look.

The point is: There's a baby in there, a baby who will do very nicely if you keep its environment snug and secure and predictable. This baby does not need its home to go crashing into a snowbank. This baby does not need the thrill of a snowmobile right now, and neither does its mother. I can't force you off the top of a mountain or off that snazzy snowmobile or off those water skis. There will always be patients who ignore their doctors' orders. But I can urge you, as strongly as possible, not to be one of them.

STRESS

No clearcut evidence exists as to the effect of stressful situations on pregnancy. Major life stresses, however, do seem to affect outcomes. This makes sense. A death in the family, for instance, can cause great anxiety, which can easily alter appetite and sleep patterns, either of which can affect the health of a pregnant woman and therefore the fetus she's carrying.

While there's often nothing anyone can do to stop the arrival of stress-inducing bad news, there might be something to be done about the stress itself. Therapy, or meditating, or having an occasional pregnancy massage, are a few options. There are special massage techniques used in pregnancy, and special equipment, too, such as a table with a "sling," where the stomach can be comfortably supported. If you're having a massage, make sure the masseur or masseuse is familiar with the special needs of pregnancy.

Another option to help relieve stress is putting off personal involvement to the extent that it's humanly possible; if you have a choice between confronting a stressful situation now and the same stressful situation later, later might make more sense. And if it *is* possible to delay a stress-inducing situation altogether—moving, for instance, or a change in career—you probably should strongly weigh benefits against risks.

TRAVEL

Patients often ask about the advisability of flying; this is a particularly big concern among working women. In terms of how you travel, I make a blanket statement, which is this: For the most part today, travel in commercial, pressurized jets is safe for pregnant women. (Well, it's as safe as it is for anyone else.) I'm less fond of the idea of island-hopping on little prop planes, because of the theoretical dramatic changes in air pressure. This could cause a problem such as premature rupture of the membranes (the amniotic sac being an enclosed space that, like many enclosed spaces, can break if subjected to sudden and extreme changes in atmospheric pressure). Some women express concern to me about the radiation exposure that occurs on flights, as well as during security checkpoints. These exposures have never been shown to be harmful to pregnant women. (If you're worried and want more specific statistics, though, you might ask to see a genetics counselor at the hospital where you'll be delivering.)

Airlines tend to be stricter on the subject of flying than doctors are. To avoid last-minute check-in nightmares— women refused admission onto planes leaving for Paris—

we make form letters available to document a patient's gestational age for the airline. Up until 34 weeks I'm usually comfortable with a woman flying. I'll ask her to stop in for a visit with me a few days prior to leaving, if she's going to be away for at least a week, but that's really more for her peace of mind than mine. I also encourage patients to get the name and number of a doctor at the destination, just in case. If she's in her third trimester, I'll also provide her with a set of her medical records, in the unlikely event that something happens while she's far from home.

I recommend that, once in the air, a patient get up and walk around during the flight. This is important; sitting in one place for too long a time can lead to leg cramps or even blood clots. Generally, though, a pregnant woman's bladder is going to feel full and she'll need to get up and walk to the bathroom anyway.

Basically, if your pregnancy is proceeding without any major problems, you should assume that you can travel, within reason. But once a problem is diagnosed, your doctor reserves the right to change your travel plans, so you might want to think about buying some travel insurance instead of outright losing your thousand-dollar round-trip ticket to Rome.

As for *where* a patient might want to travel, very rarely would I advise a woman that, based on her medical history, she shouldn't leave town. If she's traveling to a high altitude, I'll suggest that she not exercise or do anything strenuous during her stay, but altitude alone doesn't seem to affect the body's ability to oxygenate at rest. I will, however, advise against visits to Third World countries. For most of my patients, this is not a problem, but occasionally the issue does come up. Many of the immunizations are safe, but who needs the anxiety of worrying about exposure to new strains of bacteria—to say nothing of the health care available should a problem arise?

When I was pregnant I did travel a little. Jeff and I went to a beach resort for a perfectly pleasant week. But I never did *anything* that I thought might even remotely put the twins at risk. I kept out of the Jacuzzi and didn't sun-worship, and I was careful never to become overheated. It's true that I wasn't a daredevil type to begin with, but even if you are, try to accept the greater challenge right now of curtailing your impulses.

CAFFEINE

I want my patients to enjoy life as much as they can during pregnancy, and for some women life is made more enjoyable by drinking coffee or Coke. There are doctors who are absolutists, advising their patients to avoid caffeine at all costs. Studies have shown a tendency toward lower birth weight (see next section, "Smoking") among mothers who drank more than 300 mg.—or three cups—of coffee a day, but I see no problem with enjoying caffeine in moderation, which to my way of thinking means one daily eight-ounce cup.

The same holds for drinks with artificial sweeteners. If you want to have a diet soda with Nutrasweet, I give you the nod, but again I'd want you to have only one eight-ounce glass. (If you go slightly over this eight-ounces-a-day rule, you're really not going to be doing any harm, but those wily, wise grandmothers have an apt saying for this situation, too: *All things in moderation*.)

SMOKING

The question of smoking still crops up in my practice, even though we all know by now that it's definitely harmful to both mother and baby. Of course I try to get every single one of my patients to quit cold turkey. I'm a diehard anti-smoking advocate, but I also understand that it's an addiction, and that for some well-meaning women, quitting is almost impossible. If you're pregnant and still smoking, I'll say to you what I say to my pregnant patients who have packs of Merit Ultra Lights stashed in their pocketbooks, just waiting to be lit up the minute they leave my office: *If there was ever a time in your life when it was important for you to quit smoking, this is it.* But sometimes they just can't do it. I don't recommend the use of the nicotine patch at this time, but I do recommend cutting way, way down to perhaps two or three cigarettes a day, five at the very most.

These days, a pregnant woman who smokes probably has to go somewhere in secret to have her cigarette. People are very fierce when it comes to the topic; we know so much more now about the effects of smoking than we did when our mothers were pregnant. Back then, my mother smoked and drank alcohol happily throughout her pregnancy. Yes, she "got away with it," but we do know with certainty that these factors can affect fetal outcome. Your pack of Merit Ultra Lights will include a warning, in tiny typeface, that smoking can lead to—among other annoyances such as lung cancer—low birth weight in babies. Most women don't understand what "low birth weight" means. A woman who really wants to keep smoking throughout her pregnancy may rationalize to herself that "low birth weight" implies a smaller, doll-sized, but otherwise healthy baby. If that were the case, I wouldn't be urging you so strongly to kick your habit now. Low birth weight means under 5 pounds 8 ounces, or 2500 grams. These babies sometimes don't thrive; they can even have lifelong developmental problems. So you'll really want to give quitting smoking your full attention, and perhaps think about getting professional help from a behaviorist or an addiction specialist if you find it's too hard to do on your own.

ALCOHOL AND DRUGS

Not surprisingly, one of the most common concerns among first-time patients involves the use, prior and ongoing, of alcohol and drugs—prescription and/or recreational. You can't change what you've already ingested while pregnant—the Dramamine you took to get on a plane to Mexico, the bottle of wine you downed on your birthday—but there are very few situations in which the obstetrician is going to be truly alarmed by something you've done. I encourage—if only for the patient's peace of mind—full disclosure of past habits and present conditions. Let's look at the usual problem areas and address them individually.

• **Alcohol.** If you drank wine before you knew you were pregnant and now worry about the possible consequences, just remember that serious side effects such as fetal alcohol syndrome involve mothers who have consumed something closer to six drinks a day. Studies that have looked at alcohol generally have found no adverse effects for babies whose mothers have consumed up to two ounces of alcohol a day. (Two ounces is the amount that's usually in an entire drink, whether a shot of hard liquor or a glass of wine or beer.)

That said, this is certainly not the time to drink alcohol to excess, and this may well be the time not to drink at all. Most of my patients feel most comfortable giving up alcohol completely. When I was pregnant, I did have a glass of wine on a couple of occasions, including after my amniocentesis, and no doctor I know would consider this harmful. But the fact is, what you drink is what the fetus drinks; when alcohol enters your bloodstream, it enters the baby's, too. If you're like me and most women I know, you don't want to do *anything* that conceivably could harm the fetus, and while studies haven't proven that light consumption of alcohol can lead to complications, do you really want to take the chance?

If alcohol *is* that important to you, then you really should examine whether you're as moderate a drinker as you might think. Habitual consumption of alcohol can complicate a pregnancy, leading to miscarriage or premature delivery, and, some studies suggest, developmental problems throughout childhood. Excessive consumption of alcohol can lead to mental deficiency and physical deformities. Although this level of heavy drinking is not a probable scenario for most women, if it is for you, you must seek counseling immediately—for the sake of your child.

• **Over-the-counter and prescription drugs.** I think many of us are still haunted by images of Thalidomide babies from our mothers' era—children born with flipper-like appendages because of a seemingly mild and harmless drug their mothers took when pregnant. Times have changed vastly since then, and now most medications are assigned ratings by the Food and Drug Administration—A, B, C, D or X—with A being safe during pregnancy and X being truly unsafe.

Prenatal vitamins (see the "Diet" section on page 47) are given an A rating. Tylenol gets a B rating, as do all similar products that are comprised of acetaminophen, although you should double-check with your doctor before you start self-prescribing. (The reason doctors will stipulate Tylenol or some other specifically acetaminophen-containing pain reliever is that the aspirin or ibuprofen alternatives have been associated with bleeding complications.) Drugs such as Thalidomide and chemotherapy, which demonstrably lead to birth defects or other adverse outcomes, are given the forbidden rating of X. Many drugs of the sort you might be worried about—tranquilizers, anti-depressants, allergy drugs, etc.—have been given a rating of C or D. This means that studies in animals and sometimes in humans have suggested there may be potential harm if the drug is taken in pregnancy. "Potential harm" is a catchall term that pharmaceutical companies use, and, depending on the drug, it can refer to anything from a mild rash to cancer. A certain vagueness is understandable here, as there simply aren't that many studies designed to decisively determine whether a drug is reliably unsafe for pregnant humans. Still, what's important to understand is that you don't need to lose sleep over that half a Valium you once took. (By the way, no study has ever proven that diazepam [Valium] causes birth defects.)

There are many factors that need to be considered when looking at a medication, such as dose, window of exposure, and duration of exposure. Most studies look at chronic use of a drug to measure its relative safety or danger. The studies that suggest potential harm aren't referring to the woman popping a single pill, or even the woman who took the occasional anti-anxiety pill before she discovered she was pregnant. They're referring, instead, to *constant, ongoing, high-dose usage* of a drug. For the most part, it seems to require high doses of medication taken over an extended time to affect the outcome of a pregnancy.

As I've said, there are very few situations in which your obstetrician is going to be overly worried about something you've already done, but one exception is if you've already taken Accutane for acne while you were pregnant. This would be a pretty surprising event these days, as any doctor prescribing this drug knows to make sure that a patient taking it is not planning on becoming pregnant. (It can lead to central nervous system defects, undersized ears, absence of ears, and aortic abnormalities.) In the unlikely event that you have already taken a drug that might put your fetus at risk, however, you may want to discuss termination of pregnancy with your doctor—but I hasten to add that in my entire career, I have yet to personally see a situation in which a drug that a patient took has put her fetus at obvious risk.

As for drugs you might take over the remainder of your pregnancy, restrictions or recommendations differ on a case-by-case basis, so you'll need to discuss these with your doctor. Most of the drugs classified as C or D have at some point been prescribed for pregnant women; whether they should be prescribed for you is a question of weighing benefits against risks.

Sometimes a doctor can substitute one drug for another. For instance, if a patient is taking coumadin, a blood-thinner associated with known congenital anomalies, I can switch her over to heparin, which is considered safe for pregnant women. Sometimes a doctor can't make a substitution, but can still feel justified prescribing drugs that have shown *some* possibility of potential harm to the fetus. For instance, there are anti-seizure drugs with a D rating, but a seizure is something I'd obviously like to control if the attacks are of the kind that would pose a threat to the mother or her fetus. So don't be surprised or alarmed if you develop a flu or case of bronchitis during the course of your pregnancy and your doctor prescribes a medicine that contains codeine or even something stronger. Chances are your doctor has weighed the risks against the benefits and decided that it's more important for you to recover your strength.

With regard to skin flare-ups, most over-the-counter acne treatments are considered safe; generally, you're using a small amount of medication on a small area of skin. If you are under the care of a dermatologist, you might ask about a pregnancy-safe antibiotic ointment.

Some women develop oily skin and new acne in pregnancy, but others find that their skin is suddenly quite dry. Facial moisturizers are safe to use at this time.

Some other related areas of concern include:

1. *Dental visits.* Can you go to the dentist? Yes. Pregnancy is not a time to avoid dental health issues; in fact, one recent study indicates that gum disease could be linked to premature delivery. You should always alert the dentist and dental assistant to your pregnancy, and you should mention an upcoming dental visit to your obstetrician. Avoid X rays, if possible. But even oral surgery can be done with a local anesthetic, without epinephrine (more about that in a moment), and many antibiotics are safe to take during pregnancy.

2. *Antidepressants.* We live in a Prozac nation these days, and I continually encounter women who

want to know if it's safe to keep taking their antidepressants when they're pregnant. The drugs have changed their lives, they confide to me. Before Prozac and Paxil and the others, they were unhappy, perhaps even desperately so. But now they are leading fulfilling lives and are eagerly anticipating motherhood. How can they possibly give up their sense of well-being for nine months?

This is a very tricky and complex question. My feeling, again, is that if a drug isn't absolutely necessary in pregnancy, it shouldn't be given. Doctors were by and large prescribing Prozac to pregnant women without reservations until very recently, when a study in the *New England Journal of Medicine* showed a higher preterm delivery rate and a higher small-for-gestational-age rate among the babies of Prozac-taking mothers. Many doctors still prescribe Prozac to pregnant women, but now, as always happens in the wake of new studies in medical journals, they have to weigh risks and benefits.

When a patient who comes to me before getting pregnant brings her antidepressant use to my attention, I give a call to her psychiatrist or psychopharmacologist to discuss how he or she thinks this woman would fare off the drug. If it's important that the patient continue on her antidepressant, then she'll be followed closely through the pregnancy for fetal growth abnormalities. But if her prior depression wasn't life-threateningly severe and can be treated with psychotherapy, then it seems sensible to take her off the drug. A patient who stays off an antidepressant through the pregnancy can be restarted immediately after delivery when the risk of postpartum depression sets in. This will mean, however, that she may not be breastfeeding. I'm an advocate of breastfeeding (see page 221)—although with twins, I lasted only four weeks, itself no small feat—but there are times when bottle is truly better than breast, and it is up to you and your doctor to decide if this is one of them. Your baby will do fine on Similac, but your entire life may depend upon you getting your Prozac.

3. *Cold medications.* As for conditions that aren't life-threatening but are merely uncomfortable, such as the common cold, I still believe patients might be happier if given something to help them breathe freely and get a good night's sleep. An exhausted pregnant woman with a head cold who can't sleep because she's got a stuffed-up nose has a lowered resistance, leaving herself open to other, more serious respiratory ailments. If you've got a bad cold, you might want to start with something non-medicinal, such as chicken soup, tea, and a cold-steam humidifier, then add Tylenol as you need it, and, if necessary, the decongestant Sudafed or the plain version of the cough medicine Robitussin. Also be aware that Nyquil and other cold remedies contain alcohol.

4. *X rays.* These involve radiation, which can cause
   cellular change in rapidly growing tissues.
   During the first and second trimesters, fetal
   growth is so rapid that these cells are particularly vulnerable, and therefore radiation is not
   something you want to be exposed to. To the
   extent that you can avoid all X rays, you should.
   However, having issued this stern if not self-evi-
   dent warning, I can also say that sometimes X
   rays are unavoidable—and that's okay, too.

   If you had X rays before you knew you were
   pregnant, don't get hysterical. There are several
   possibilities. Did you wear a lead shield? Did it
   cover your pelvic area? Were they dental X rays,
   and therefore far from the anatomical site of the
   pregnancy? Whatever the circumstances, while
   it is likely that no harm was done, any exposure
   to an X ray definitely deserves a mention to your
   obstetrician.

   If you do happen to need X rays while pregnant—because of a fall, or due to any other medical emergency—you may notice a huge sign
   near the X ray machine reminding pregnant
   women to alert the technician about their condition. This is another of those situations where
   you (and your doctor, presumably) will need to
   weigh risks and benefits. Again, the lead shield
   will need to cover your abdomen and pelvic area;
   again, why take a chance unless it's absolutely
   necessary?

   As for dental X rays: As mentioned earlier in
   this section, this is no time to avoid dental care;

but, as I just stressed, this *is* a time to avoid radiation, if possible. Therefore, see your dentist, but postpone elective X rays until after the pregnancy.

• **Recreational drugs.** After you've confessed the occasional Valium or glass of wine to your doctor, you still may have some concerns that are slightly less easy to discuss: recreational drugs. If you smoked marijuana before you knew you were pregnant, I don't think you should worry. The conclusions that have been drawn about the effects of marijuana in pregnancy have mostly centered on a lowered fertility rate which, at least in your situation, isn't a pressing problem.

The links that have been established between cocaine use in the mother and such problems as learning deficits and even addictions in children primarily exist in situations where there has been chronic usage. Chronic cocaine use is also associated with high blood pressure, which leads to poor perfusion (passage of blood between mother and fetus), which in turn can lead to premature separation of the placenta from the uterine wall—also known as *abruptio placenta*. This is a life-threatening condition for both mother and baby.

Of course, now that you know you're pregnant, any use of recreational drugs should stop, period. If you have any concerns about drugs you've taken, you should certainly be upfront with your doctor. And if you don't feel that you can discuss these worries—well, then, you've chosen the wrong doctor.

SEXUALLY TRANSMITTED DISEASES

Sex is one area where your past behavior might affect the health of the baby. Even in the unlikely event that this was the case, however, finger-pointing and guilt-mongering would be counterproductive. The focus at this time should be on how to help yourself, and how to help your baby.

• **Hepatitis B.** This is checked in the first blood test to rule out chronic carrier state. If the blood test determines that the patient does indeed fit this profile, it means that her body fluids are infectious and that there is the risk of transmission to the baby. Newborns will receive protection in the form of hepatitis B vaccine and a special immunoglobulin.

• **Syphilis.** Also checked in the first blood test, syphilis can be associated with fetal abnormalities of the teeth, bones, and central nervous system. Simple penicillin administered to a pregnant woman has been shown to reduce the risk to the baby.

• **Chlamydia and gonorrhea.** If you've been treated for any other sexually transmitted disease, then you should be screened for gonorrhea and chlamydia. In both cases, the diagnosis is determined through cultures of the cervix. Both flare up intermittently, often after years of dormancy, so it's difficult to know whether they'll be active as the baby passes through the birth canal. They're both treatable by antibiotics but just to be safe, antibiotic ointment is applied to the newborn's eyes in the delivery room.

• **Genital warts.** These are caused by human papilloma virus, or hPV. In the most extreme cases—among immuno-compromised women, such as those with HIV-positive status—genital warts can manifest themselves as large cauliflower lesions. In these situations, the warts can be excised or frozen off, but we wouldn't use acids to remove them from pregnant women. As for small genital warts, these don't play a major role in pregnancies, though sometimes obstetricians remove them during delivery, while an anesthetic is already in place.

• **Herpes simplex virus.** This is a sexually transmitted infection associated with genital ulcers. The first outbreak is often severe and painful; recurrences are milder. If an outbreak occurs close to delivery, it could be catastrophic for the baby, who might contract it from an active genital lesion while passing through the birth canal. In those instances, the baby would be delivered by cesarean section to dramatically decrease the risk of exposure. Recurrent outbreaks carry a much lower risk of transmission to the baby, because the mother would have developed antibodies. However, most of us still recommend delivery by cesarean section if there is *any* active genital lesion at the time of labor.

• **HIV.** Testing for HIV status is mandated on a state-by-state basis. In New York State, we must offer testing to all pregnant women, and all newborns are automatically tested. Whether a patient agrees to be tested or not, she will learn the results of the newborn's test. If a patient declines to be tested, she has to sign a form declaring that she was informed of her options, that she understands the risks and benefits, and that she refuses. Of course, we urge our patients to undergo the test; if ever there was a time to find out whether you're HIV positive, this is it. And lately we've been able to add a persuasive element to our argument: Recent studies clearly show that the use of AZT during pregnancy and delivery can significantly decrease the risk of transmission of HIV to the baby.

SEX

Pregnancy, of course, is a time of seismically profound hormonal changes. Inevitably, these will affect your sex life. While some women experience a diminished sex drive, others find themselves feeling more sexual than ever. Don't be surprised to find yourself at one extreme or the other, depending on the stage of your pregnancy.

But physical factors aren't the only ones that might affect your sex drive. Fear and anxiety play a significant role too, for both the man and the woman. The man sometimes feels that he's going to hurt the baby if he thrusts too hard during intercourse, and the whole experience has a walking-on-eggshells quality that doesn't make for anybody's idea of great sex. Then again, the absence of birth control can lead to a more carefree environment. Women often experience a greater sense of freedom, especially during the second trimester, when any morning sickness has probably passed, the pregnancy is well-established, and the exhaustion has lifted.

There are some conditions in which sex is definitely not allowed. If a patient who has begun bleeding comes to me in the first trimester, I always tell her to abstain from sexual intercourse until there's been no bleeding for a week. Again, this falls under the common sense category.

Another situation in which I would strongly advise abstinence is placenta previa. This refers to the condition in which the placenta overlaps the cervix. This is not a problem in the first trimester, and is often first detected on routine ultrasound in the second trimester. Most women will have no symptoms associated with a placenta previa, but occasionally a woman will bleed in the second or third trimester.

In the three-dimensional structure of the uterine cavity, the placenta has to implant somewhere, and chances are that somewhere will be on the "roof" or the "wall." But in placenta previa, it happens to be on the "floor" of the uterus, and covers the cervix, blocking the baby's potential exit. This isn't an uncommon diagnosis at early stages of the pregnancy, but nearly all of these cases will resolve on their own by term—among first-time mothers, the incidence rate at delivery is one in 250. Until such a case is resolved, however, I'll put the woman on what is genteelly called "pelvic rest" (mentioned briefly in Chapter 2)—which is another way of saying "no intercourse"—because the placenta is at increased risk for trauma in that location.

What about other kinds of less invasive sex—oral sex and masturbation? With your doctor's permission (and a doctor usually wouldn't restrict a patient's sex life during most of the pregnancy) these activities pose no threat to the fetus. As I noted in Chapter 2, the labia undergo significant changes during pregnancy that might give a sensation of genital pressure; this won't necessarily translate into desire, often just discomfort.

Oral sex is safe. We know that the vagina is the furthest thing in the world from a sterile environment, but we also know that neither oral sex nor intercourse (nor, for that matter, taking a bath or swimming) breaks down the barrier between the uterus and the world. As I noted in Chapter 2, however, pregnancy can cause vaginal secretions to become heavier, which may affect your partner's enjoyment of oral sex.

Masturbation is safe, too, but in any of these cases if the sex leads to an orgasm, you should be aware that during climax pregnant women often feel a more intense than usual wave of feeling that can even include a few brief moments of cramping—a kind of mini-contraction. This is normal. It may not be entirely pleasant, and you may not want to repeat the experience, but do not become frightened if it happens, or, later in the pregnancy, think that you've gone into labor. (Remember that actual, real labor is a big deal, and usually doesn't just "happen" out of nowhere. The only situation where this advice does *not* hold true is if there are risk factors for preterm labor, in which case even small contractions may be enough to cause cervical change. But we're getting ahead of ourselves. For more on the subject, see Chapter 8.) Mini-contractions triggered by orgasm are *much, much, much* weaker and less defined than anything you will experience in labor. So feel free to masturbate and have oral sex and make love to your heart's content.

Or feel just as free not to.

All women are different; it's hard to tell where you will fall on the spectrum of sex drive. In my experience, though, the typical pregnant woman wants to abstain from sex for most of the pregnancy.

I did have sex during pregnancy, and even though I knew I had nothing to worry about, an apprehension was present, which made our sex less carefree than it might have been. So maybe it wasn't the most sexually active time of my life, but I don't think either of us really cared. Our bodies could do what they liked, but our minds, to tell the truth, were elsewhere.

the
second
trimester

Chapter Five
The Calm

- Whether to Test
- Ultrasound
- Triple screen
- Amniocentesis

The second trimester of a pregnancy is actually a very low-key time, in terms of both a doctor's work and a pregnant woman's point of view. Much of this trimester is taken up by what I consider fluff, at least relative to the other two trimesters. Sometimes I don't really know what to do to fill up a patient's entire visit. Other than weighing her, checking her urine, taking her blood pressure, listening to a heartbeat and assessing the fundal height, there's not all that much for us to do, and we end up talking a little bit about what movies we've seen. Many of the big discussions have been taken care of in the first couple of visits.

The second trimester has been described as the wonderful rest in the middle of a long trek, or the calm in the middle of a storm. You've weathered the sometimes difficult early days, and you've passed the point of most of the valid miscarriage worries. What you're left with is often a period of well-being, in which many of the rough edges such as morning sickness and intense breast tenderness have been smoothed over. Many women in the second trimester take new pleasure in the way they feel and look; the body is filling out, the stomach is growing larger, and the fullness begins to feel more natural, as though they've always looked and felt this way.

Which is not to say that the second trimester lacks drama. On the contrary, this is also a period in which important tests may be done, tests which may lead to further decisions—tests which I happen to have very strong feelings about.

WHETHER TO TEST

Aside from non-optional screens such as the one for gestational diabetes, there are three procedures that I offer in the coming weeks: a sonogram, a triple-screen blood test, and an amniocentesis. I'll have already discussed these with a patient at one of the first visits, in order to give her plenty of opportunities to consider her options. But by the second trimester, the time has come either to schedule the tests or not. She has to reach some decisions now—and that says something about a growing fetus's relentless march toward maturity. There's no cure for procrastination like a pregnancy.

I'll discuss each of these procedures in great detail later in this chapter, but first, as I do with many of my patients, I'd like to take this opportunity to clear the air. Sometimes when I raise the question of any one of these tests, the patient will interrupt and say: "I don't need that. I'll take my chances." Or: "I don't want to know, because we wouldn't do anything about it anyway." And then I'll respond: "You know, we're not necessarily talking about termination."

"Take my chances," "do something about it," "termination": What we're all really talking about—or, perhaps, talking *around*—is abortion. I think it might help if we come right out and name the issue that's at the back of many people's minds whenever the question of second-trimester testing arises. I firmly believe in a woman's right to choose—but that doesn't necessarily mean the choice will be to abort a genetically questionable fetus, or a fetus with a structural abnormality. For some women, it means the right to choose to keep the fetus, no matter what a test might show. It's a patient's legal right to choose, and it's my job to help her see that choice through to the end, whatever that may be. And, like most obstetricians, I do hear the full gamut of viewpoints. I have patients who tell me, "Listen, it's not an easy decision to make, but there's *no way* we could deal with a Down syndrome baby." Then again, I have patients who say to me, "The rabbi says, 'No testing!'"

Either way, I think it's important for you to know that there are *two* issues at stake when it comes to second-trimester testing. One, indeed, is ethical. But the other is medical.

What I tell my patients is true: We're *not* necessarily talking about termination. There are reasons other than possibly ending the pregnancy for finding out everything you can about the development of the fetus—sound medical reasons that you should at least consider before deciding whether to pursue a particular test. Those reasons are different for each of these three tests (I'll get to those reasons soon), and indeed I don't necessarily recommend all three tests for everyone. But in general, my feeling about what these tests reveal is the same as for almost all medical information: the more, the better.

The information is *out there*. It exists, and it's easily available, for the most part. And thanks to dramatic break-throughs in genetic testing that seem to come along every year or so, more and more information is available all the time. So why not get it?

If a test indicates an abnormality—either a possibility of one, or a certainty—then we know to monitor the situation. This might mean closer observation of the patient; maybe it means more testing to confirm the preliminary results. It could call for nothing more than the doctor flagging your chart; then again, it might mean scheduling a pediatric specialist to be present at the birth, rather than having to page one frantically as a routine delivery suddenly develops into a full-blown emergency that puts both child and mother at risk.

What's more, this extra information might help *you*, by encouraging you to seek counseling in advance—for instance, joining a support group for parents of Down syndrome children—so that you're able to welcome your new baby in the best of psychological health. This, in turn, will inevitably help both you *and* your child.

And then there's always the possibility that a patient will change her mind. What once seemed unthinkable can turn acceptable when the theoretical becomes reality. In my experience over the years, I've seen it happen to even the most ardent of abortion opponents.

For the most part, I can convince a patient to at least consider the testing. But in the end, of course, it's her decision.

Now, sometimes this information doesn't come without costs, financial or otherwise. Just the other day, I saw a patient who didn't have insurance, but I still strongly recommended that she have certain tests, such as a second-trimester ultrasound and relevant genetic screening. As someone who has seen how quickly the bills from a pregnancy can mount, I'm more than empathetic—but as a doctor who has witnessed my share of grief and suffering, I'm also more than emphatic about the importance of these tests.

The tests can also take a certain emotional toll. A false positive can raise concerns that make everyone worried and eventually lead to nothing, and you'll wind up feeling that you could have lived without all that extra anxiety. But from a medical point of view, I feel it's important to educate yourself as thoroughly as science and reason will allow.

What's essential here, and what I really can't emphasize enough, is that two patients receiving the same information might well reach different decisions—but at least they'll be basing their decisions on all the information that medical science has made available. As you read about these three tests, and as you discuss them with your own obstetrician, I ask only that you remember this: The more information you have, the better equipped you'll be to arrive at decisions that are right for *you*.

ULTRASOUND

If I had to pick the one test that a second-trimester patient should have, this is it: the anatomical ultrasound, also known as a sonogram.

If you haven't had an ultrasound yet, now's a great time, if only to make sure you're not carrying multiple fetuses. And whether or not you've had one earlier in the pregnancy, this is an excellent opportunity to check on fetal development. The American College of Obstetricians and Gynecologists doesn't advocate ultrasonography on what's commonly called a routine basis, citing cost-benefit studies, but I disagree. Cost-benefit studies certainly have their usefulness, but they base their calculations on broad economic principles pertaining to all of society, not to the medical needs of a specific patient.

Ultrasonography has also recently come under attack for its supposed unreliability. Again, I have to disagree. True, ultrasounds can and do produce false positives and false negatives, even in the best hands using the best equipment —but this technique still provides the best information available. When it comes down to a patient sitting across from me in my office, I can't think of a single good reason why she'd want to skip an anatomical ultrasound. It can be immensely helpful from a medical point of view, reassuring from a psychological point of view, and it carries virtually zero risk.

This test is performed roughly mid-trimester, which is to say anywhere from the 18th through the 20th week. While nearly all prenatal testing can be done in the obstetrician's office, this is one exam for which I strongly recommend you find an expert. I saw a perinatologist for my anatomical ultrasound, and that's the kind of specialist I'd send you to see. There are also skilled radiologists with specialized training in perinatal ultrasound. (If you're having an amniocentesis, you'll also be having an ultrasound at the same time. More about that later in this chapter.)

The anatomical ultrasound differs from the basic first-trimester ultrasound you might have undergone at an earlier date, in that it's far more thorough. In addition to verifying the number of fetuses and their viability, the doctor will also survey the amount of amniotic fluid, the position of the placenta, and will determine whether the umbilical cord attaches to the middle or the side of the placenta (the middle facilitates better fetal growth). Then the focus shifts to the fetal structures: the cerebellum, the diameter and shape of the head, the spine (vertebra by vertebra), the lengths of the arm bones and leg bones, a four-chambered view of the heart, the stomach, the bladder and kidneys, the insertion of the umbilical cord into the abdomen, the abdominal wall, the genitalia. (If you don't want to know the sex of the fetus, it's important that you tell the sonographer in advance.)

A skilled sonographer will also be able to check the position of the feet, the number of digits on the hands and feet, the profile of the face, the lips and nose, and the distance between the eyes. All this information, in turn, will help determine whether the gestational age previously arrived at is correct, and whether the fetus is growing appropriately.

As you might expect from something called an anatomical ultrasound, this test is also useful in detecting structural malformations (birth defects). These can range from such extreme cases as anencephaly (in which all or part of the upper brain and skull are missing) and hydrocephaly (accumulated fluid on the brain), to more subtle (but perhaps equally serious) malformations such as heart defects, skeletal abnormalities, and neural tube defects, as well as facial clefts and hernias.

If you haven't undergone one earlier, you should understand that an ultrasound is a noninvasive look at the fetus on a monitor that resembles a small TV screen. Some doctors ask their patients to drink a lot of water before this test (to help aid visualization), but I don't think that's necessary; by this point in the pregnancy, in fact, you don't want a full bladder getting in the way of the view. The doctor or technician applies ultrasound conducting gel (warm, I hope) onto your bare abdomen, then takes something called a transducer, which is about the size and shape of a microphone, and moves it along the surface of your stomach. As he or she does this, sound waves are emitted and bounced back to the transducer and interpreted, producing an image of the fetus.

I have performed ultrasounds countless times, and yet each time a fetus appears, I feel a shiver of recognition and vicarious excitement. As the fetus is viewed, various "snapshots" are taken—stills that are used in measuring and assessing its development. Usually, the mother is given a couple of these to take home. Although the technology is improving, these photos might not bear much of a resemblance to a baby, but there they are: the first snapshots for the baby book.

TRIPLE SCREEN

This is a simple blood test, performed in the obstetrician's office, that measures three hormone levels: alpha-fetoprotein (AFP), human chorionic gonadotropin (hCG), and unconjugated estriol. These three serum markers together can offer risk assessments for various abnormalities, and it's worth your while to understand what each marker tells us.*

The test generally takes place at 15 to 20 weeks. For a patient with a history of genetic disorders, I'd perform the

---

*A word to those of you carrying multiples: Serum screens are not as useful in your case, so you need to discuss the risk of chromosomal abnormalities with your doctor.

test as early as possible, at the 15th or 16th week. The principle behind the testing is this: Whatever is in the amniotic sac fluid inevitably passes into the mother's bloodstream, so the blood sample that's drawn from the mother's arm will contain hormones produced by the fetus. To distinguish this from fluid drawn directly from the amniotic sac in an amniocentesis, this is usually called maternal serum AFP, or MSAFP.

If the MSAFP level is elevated (and you'd hear from your doctor with this news within one or two days), the fetus has an increased risk of a neural tube defect (NTD) or an abdominal wall defect (gastroschisis or omphalocele). An NTD results from the failure of the neural tube to close in the early stages of development, and it can signify such malformations as anencephaly, which is fatal, or spina bifida (open spine), which can be severely debilitating. While a family history of NTD in either parent increases the risk for the child, it's important to remember that the vast majority—some nine out of 10 cases—happen among the offspring of parents without such histories.

If the MSAFP level is low, the fetus has an increased risk of Down syndrome or other, even more severe chromosomal abnormalities. A child with Down syndrome will exhibit varying degrees of mental retardation and a characteristic round, flat facial type, and will be at risk for congenital heart disease, gastrointestinal problems, and childhood leukemias. While the statistical risk of having a Down syndrome child increases with the mother's age, the majority—about four out of five cases—happen among women under the arbitrary "advanced maternal age" of 35.

(Down syndrome, which is caused by Trisomy 21—meaning an extra copy of chromosome number 21—is the most common genetic abnormality seen at term, occurring in one out of 800 live births, so it's not unreasonable to cite it as a possible adverse outcome. I'll stick to that tradition here, with this caveat: Down syndrome ranges in degree, and does not preclude a meaningful, fulfilling life.)

For many years, only AFP was measured. More recently, we've learned that measurements from two other markers can also be indicative of Down syndrome and other abnormalities: elevated levels of hCG and low levels of unconjugated estriol. Alone, AFP will detect about one out of four cases of Down syndrome; when all three markers are evaluated together, the detection rate more than doubles. Therefore I always recommend triple screens to my patients.

As I've said, the triple screen doesn't give a conclusive diagnosis. In fact, the false-positive rate is very high. Of the abnormal readings, approximately 99 percent are eventually determined to be false positives. When a triple screen comes back with an abnormal result, the obstetrician should call the patient immediately, sounding appropriate alarms but also offering appropriate reassurances. All the results mean so far is that further testing is necessary.

When the MSAFP is elevated, we repeat the blood test. A normal level the second time around would cancel out the first reading, which might have been due to a small amount of blood exchanged between mother and fetus, during a first-trimester bleed, for instance. A second high MSAFP, however, would call for further testing, as would one low MSAFP.

The next step would be a sonogram, both to confirm the gestational age and to rule out multiple fetuses. Since the levels of the various hormones change throughout the pregnancy, and since they're being compared to the levels that are normal at a given gestational age, an abnormality in the MSAFP testing could be due to something as simple as a miscalculation of the date of conception. Then again, it might be due to the presence of twins or triplets, which would double or triple the hormone levels.

Assuming that the gestational age was calculated correctly and that the uterus isn't housing multiple fetuses, however, the next step would be to consider an amniocentesis. At this point, I would urge the patient and her partner to attend a genetics counseling session prior to the amniocentesis so that risks, benefits, and alternatives could be fully discussed. (Again, more about amnios later in this chapter.) Then, if the amnio proceeds, and if it comes back normal, I'd still flag the chart; those earlier elevated MSAFP readings didn't come from nowhere, and might still signal something important—if not a birth defect, then maybe some manageable complication down the line, such as intrauterine growth retardation (IUGR) or early delivery. (For more on IUGR, see page 136.) Come the third trimester, I might perform more testing (a non-stress test [NST], for instance; see page 138), and another sonogram to assure fetal well-being.

If the amnio comes back abnormal, however, with an abnormal level of AFP in the fluid or with abnormal chromosomes, then we've entered a new stage of discussion. This is never easy, and can involve highly specialized genetic testing, ultrasound, and counseling.

This may sound like a lot of testing, and I can't honestly say that it doesn't sometimes become time-consuming and expensive while ultimately proving nothing. True, the triple screen carries a substantial possibility of false-positive results, and true, this contingency can be costly both financially and emotionally, especially if it leads to equally or ever-more-costly follow-up tests. The conventional wisdom seems to be that these risks outweigh the benefits. In Great Britain, where the neural-tube defect rate is approximately five or six per 1,000, the medical establishment's policy on triple-screening is to offer it to everyone. But here in the United States, where the neural-tube defect rate is less than half that of Great Britain, the screening isn't deemed "cost-effective" for patients without a family history of neural-tube defects—this despite the fact that screenings can detect 85 percent of fetuses affected by NTD.

As both patient and doctor, I was and am uncomfortable with not availing myself of every opportunity to learn about a possible complication. Each of these three serum markers has a certain sensitivity and specificity, and, as I've mentioned, the overall usefulness is improved when the test results are combined. AFP alone has a 25 percent detection rate for Down syndrome, but put all three together and the detection rate soars to approximately 60 percent. By combining serum testing with an ultrasound performed by a specialist, the rate probably nears 80 percent. That's an overall improvement in the detection rate from, roughly, one out of four to four out of five. Now, that's obviously not foolproof; ideally, you'd want a 100 percent detection rate on everything. But only an amniocentesis, which is widely considered the "gold standard" of Down syndrome detection, comes closest to offering that level of assurance.

Moreover, as I noted a few paragraphs back, even when an abnormal triple screen is followed by a normal amnio, the first, unfavorable result can still be useful as a possible warning sign of problems to come. Not only can it happen—it happened to me. When I was pregnant my test came back with an MSAFP level that was high even for a woman carrying twins. The ultrasound and amnio showed nothing out of the ordinary, but in the end I suffered what's called preterm premature rupture of the membranes (translation: My water broke too soon, before I reached term and before labor was imminent), and then I underwent preterm delivery—which is one of the possible adverse outcomes that an elevated MSAFP can suggest, even if the amnio is normal. In retrospect, I can't say I was completely surprised by these complications, considering the abnormal MSAFP in the middle of the second trimester.

AMNIOCENTESIS

Most patients assume their doctors will tell them if they should have an amnio. Most patients are wrong.

The fact is, most doctors go by the numbers alone. There are two problems with this approach. One, the numbers don't always mean what they seem to mean. Two, the numbers don't always mean what they seem to mean for *you*.

The number that comes up most often—a statistic you've probably already read or heard about—is one out of 200. That's the across-the-board risk of losing the fetus as a result of complications stemming from this procedure. Traditional wisdom holds that this risk should be balanced against the odds of finding out that the fetus has a chromosomal abnormality, a percentage that rises with age. Amniocentesis does not detect structural abnormalities— that's the purpose of the ultrasound—but it allows determination of chromosomal number and pattern. This is why it's useful in detecting Down syndrome, for example, as well as other chromosomal disorders such as Turner's syndrome (which involves the loss of an X chromosome) and Klinefelter's syndrome (which involves an extra X chromosome).

(Patients often ask if there are ever inaccuracies in an amnio report—a finding of Down syndrome or some other disorder when in fact the baby is normal, or, conversely, a normal report with a baby later found to be affected. My geneticist friend says that although it is theoretically possible, due to a mixup in the lab, she has never seen or heard of such an instance. Therefore, this is not a complication worth worrying about.)

In a study done in the 1980s among amnios performed in the second trimester, the risk equaled the benefit—the numbers matched, one out of 200—at the age of 35. But that, as they say, was then. By now, of course, technology has made a decade's worth of progress, and it stands to reason that the risks associated with performing this procedure have decreased. Yet even though the one-in-200 statistic is hopelessly out of date, it endures to this day, affecting the official policies of thousands of medical and insurance organizations and the decisions of millions of pregnant women.

What's more, even if the number were still accurate, it might not apply to your individual circumstances. If you were my patient, for instance, the ultrasound equipment guiding your amniocentesis would not only be far more advanced than what it was ten years ago, it very likely would be more advanced than what's available at many other hospitals. It's always being updated, and it's always state-of-the-art. This means that there is very accurate visualization during the amnio, allowing us to gain access to the amniotic fluid without passing through the placenta or the umbilical cord (and thereby allowing us to decrease the risk of the procedure).

And then there are the people who are assisting during the procedure. I perform all my amnio procedures at the hospital, with the assistance of the staff there. Because of the high volume of patients at this teaching hospital, a patient getting an amnio or ultrasound under these circumstances has to be on the above-average end of the statistical spectrum.

And chances are, so are you. You might not know where you fall statistically, but if you're reading this book, you're a woman who wants good care, and assuming you've placed yourself in experienced hands, that's what you're probably getting.

So here's the advice I offer patients when they start talking numbers: *Throw the numbers out.*

It's simply not a valid way to reach a decision. Instead, I tell them that they need to sit down with their partners and discuss what they want to know, and what they would do based on what they might find out.

So what will you want to consider? While the old statistics no longer apply, the risk/benefit trade-off is a valid way to think about it. Increased maternal age is indeed linked with certain genetic abnormalities, the most common of which is Down syndrome. I think all women need to understand that the risks of carrying a child with Down syndrome do go up with age, and that statistics clearly bear this out.

Are you over 35? That's an easy one: Have the test. Like it or not, you've reached what we call AMA—advanced maternal age. If you're 31 to 34, you're borderline AMA. And if you're 30 or younger, you're not in a high-risk group. But remember: Even if you're not yet old enough to vote, you're only in a low-risk group, not a *no*-risk group. There's no such thing as a zero chance of having a baby with a serious genetic abnormality. No matter what your age, you'll still need to make a decision.

I do this sort of counseling all the time. I don't know how many times I've told a 26-year-old, or a 32-year-old, or a 22-year-old, that she needs to sit and think what it would mean to have a Down syndrome baby. Has she had any experience, positive or negative, with anyone who has Down syndrome?

Personally, I had not a doubt in my mind that I would have an amnio—and I was not yet 35. No matter how difficult it had been to achieve pregnancy (and I had quite a difficult time!), my experience as a doctor had shown me again and again how foolish I would be to think I was not at risk. And my husband, Jeff, agreed. And we also agreed that we might terminate the pregnancy in the face of a major abnormality. And, in the end, we agreed that the benefit of knowing what we wanted to know outweighed the risk of undergoing an invasive procedure.

And it *is* an invasive procedure. The obstetrician is putting a needle in your abdomen that penetrates your uterus, where it will draw out a sample of amniotic fluid. The obstetrician will be able to watch the needle on the ultrasound and therefore avoid the fetus, but the warning is worth repeating: This is an invasive procedure. The uterus is your fetus's home, and a foreign object is entering it. No matter how good the equipment, or how expert the obstetrician, such a procedure can't help but carry some risk of fetal loss.

Now, in case I've scared you, let me hurriedly offer this reassuring thought: Am I nervous when I perform an amnio? No. For most obstetricians, amnios simply come with the territory. But if for some reason you suspect your doctor is nervous or inexperienced, get one who isn't. Stop the procedure, inform the doctor that you're not comfortable, and if he or she can't offer you the proper reassurances, apologize and request a substitute. In fact, it's worth traveling to a major medical center, if that's what it takes to get someone with a sufficient level of experience. I've had patients ask me if I've ever done an amnio before, and I may be tempted to answer, "You mean today?" but I'm never insulted. I've performed hundreds of amnios, but I consider such curiosity on the part of the mother to be healthy, a way of protecting the fetus and preserving her own peace of mind. So don't be afraid to err on the side of insulting the doctor; better a wounded ego than a damaged pregnancy.

I wish I could tell you that the amnio is entirely painless. In theory, we could anesthetize the skin, but the injection of anesthetic would itself hurt, so we bypass this step (just as we would for a vaccination). We can't anesthetize your entire uterus, however, and that's where the pain comes in. The gauge of the needle—its diameter—is no wider than it would be to draw blood from your arm, but when the needle reaches its target, the uterus contracts. It's a short, sharp, shooting pain—let's put the emphasis on *short*— and, frankly, my own experience under the needle has changed the way I counsel patients. I used to tell women that the shot'll be over before they know it, which is true. But now I add that it very well might hurt.

The textbooks say that the hole in the uterine membrane will heal in a day or so. I agree that you can resume normal activities the next day, but I would add that you should avoid strenuous activity for a week—running for a bus, exercise, sex, picking up the kids, etc. You should also tell your obstetrician immediately about bleeding, fluid leak-age, or anything else out of the ordinary. And—I don't think it's just me—you'll probably experience soreness or even slight bruising at the site where the needle went in.

But you might take comfort from this: You're halfway home. While of course you'll be metaphorically biting your nails until the results come in, the amnio is a real mile-stone. I routinely suggest that a patient have half a glass of wine when she gets home from her amnio, if she wants. (I did.) The use of alcohol has been shown to have a relaxing effect on the uterus. At the very least, put your feet up—lit-erally. Not only have you earned it, but it'll help the healing. That's what I did, too. I made sure my calendar would be clear after my amnio, and when I got home, I put up my feet and had a drink. Then I picked up the baby name book for the first time, and I read it from first page to last.

Chapter Six
Enormous Changes

- •Fetal Movement
- •More Physical Changes
- •Risk of Prematurity

Once the drama of testing has passed, and assuming that your results are satisfactory, you'll be able to congratulate yourself on a job well done thus far. Your doctor may tell you that everything looks great, and in fact you probably still feel pretty great, too. But perhaps the biggest bonus of the second trimester—the greatest incentive to keep knocking back the milk and the horse-pills and the leafy greens—is the moment when you first feel a kick.

FETAL MOVEMENT

No description can do justice to this event. It tends to take place somewhere between 18 and 20 weeks for first-time mothers (sometimes earlier for veterans of maternity), though it's certainly no cause for concern if it doesn't happen exactly on schedule. (My own moment of truth came at 22 weeks.)

The sensation of an actual tiny person kicking inside you is a little like an alien inhabitation, and a little like falling in love. I never did get used to it. Sometimes when I was relaxing, putting my feet up and being a good patient, I'd feel movement and I'd shout to my husband, "Did you *see* that?"

"I can't believe you're so excited," he answered me once. "Don't you see this every day?"

I do, of course, but nothing prepared me for the real thing. I'd always asked patients, "Is the baby active? Do you feel fetal movement?" but now I *got it*. One patient described the first signs of movement—what we call "quickening"—as being vaguely aquatic. It was as though, she said, she had a little dolphin swimming around inside her, playfully turning somersaults. This is fairly accurate, when you think about it; the fetus's environment *is* aquatic, and the movements are made while suspended in fluid. Sometimes there's a smoothness to the kicks (which may not be kicks at all, but arms flailing or a head nodding), a sensation of the fetus gliding from one place to another in its watery home. The movement can be painful or uncomfortable if the fetus presses against a nerve or, as the pregnancy progresses, against the kidneys or liver, but mostly the sensation is foreign yet deeply pleasurable. Later on, when the baby gets very big, you'll often see a bump rising on the surface of your abdomen—a knee? an elbow?—as the baby moves. Enjoy your baby's movements, and as you do you'll probably start to visualize him or her more easily.

Yet as tranquil as this period is, glitches can still arise. If you should experience any of them, try to keep things in perspective. You should know that very few pregnancies are entirely problem-free. Perhaps you were planning on having the "perfect" pregnancy—working right up until the zero hour, then delivering without any fetal monitoring or pain relief—but try not to be terribly disappointed if it doesn't turn out exactly that way. There's usually some sort of problem in a pregnancy, whether it's a bit of minor spotting early on or elevated blood pressure or a sudden complication during delivery. It's helpful to realize that obstetricians expect these glitches, and that we're prepared for them. Complications can be frightening for pregnant women, but in virtually every case, we doctors have seen them before, and the majority of the time we know exactly how to treat them.

MORE PHYSICAL CHANGES

By now most of the early, unpleasant sensations of pregnancy have passed—the fatigue and nausea—and for a while, you'll probably experience smooth sailing on calm amniotic waters. Still, the physical changes never really let up, and often the first indications of what's to come are new aches and pains, such as:

• **Round ligament pains.** The round ligaments hold the uterus in its anatomical location. When you're not pregnant, your uterus is smaller than a pear. Forgive the mixed metaphor involving fruit and office supplies, but the round ligaments are like rubber bands that stretch dramatically as the formerly pearlike uterus lifts up and out of the pelvis.

Round ligament pains, which most of my patients experience at one time or another, feel like a stitch or a pull, the kind of sharp jab you sometimes feel in your side after running. I was startled myself by the sudden intensity of these pains when I had them for the first time, and I can easily understand why some women feel truly frightened and even fear that they've gone into premature labor.

Most typically, one side aches more than the other. Though you may describe these pains as sharp, even stabbing, they are completely normal. I tell my patients to do what I did, which is to soak for a while in a warm tub (*not* a Jacuzzi).

• **Showing.** Even before the lower abdomen starts to protrude, you may swear that none of your clothes fit. This, like so much in pregnancy, is due to your body's increased production of progesterone, which contributes to a bloating sensation. (The progesterone will also continue to weaken your ankles and knees, and just when you need them more than ever! Likewise, even though the nausea has probably stopped, the indigestion caused by the reflux—caused by the weakening of the esophageal sphincter, caused by— yes!—progesterone—will become more pronounced, especially as the expanding uterus pushes the stomach upward toward the esophagus.) As the uterus lifts up and out of the pelvis, it eases pressure on the bladder, and, as I've mentioned earlier, most pregnant women experience a second-trimester decrease in the frequent need to urinate.

The pigmentation changes that began in the first trimester also continue here, and you'll probably notice a dark line (or linea nigra) down the middle of your abdomen, as well as, at least in some women, a butterfly-like pattern on the face (melasma, also known as "the mask of pregnancy").

Somewhere around 20 weeks, the uterus reaches the navel, which, in most women, pops, although it's completely normal if it doesn't.

• **Backache.** This is one of the most common problems of pregnancy, and while there are some specific adjustments you can make to minimize backaches, I'm afraid that this affliction simply seems to come with the territory. After all, your body is being given an extra burden to carry. As I mentioned earlier, your ankle and knee ligaments have weakened, while at the same time the joints of your pelvis have become more lax, preparing the way for delivery. Pregnant women, whose bodies and sense of balance have altered dramatically, sometimes overcompensate in ways that make back problems even worse.

Much of the strain of a pregnancy falls specifically on the lower back. The muscles located there, which are called the paraspinous muscles, connect from one vertebra to the next. No matter what kind of shape you're in, those muscles have never quite gotten the daily workout they're getting now. Here are some backsaving tips, although they're by no means miracle cures:

1. *Stretch.* Just two to five minutes of limbering up can help keep the paraspinous muscles loose and prevent them from going into spasm. So touch those toes. Reach for the sky. (And no, there's no truth to those old wives' tales about the dangers of a pregnant woman lifting her arms above her head.)

2. *Take warm baths, or shower with a massaging shower head*—though neither will completely eliminate the discomfort.

3. *Never lift any objects without first bending your knees.*

4. *Avoid lifting heavy objects in general.* (But I think you already know that.)

5. *Wear smart, practical shoes.* You don't need to buy orthopedic lace-ups, but you should see the Imelda Marcos–meets–Manolo Blahnik numbers some of my patients totter in on. I've witnessed pregnant women in their ninth month attempting to walk across a room in stiletto spikes. This is not only bad for the back, it's dangerous to the baby, if the woman should take a tumble. Personally, I wouldn't venture much higher than an inch or two off the ground.

Your posture is clearly changing now. I know I sound like your mother, but try to remember not to hunch your shoulders. Some of my patients claim to have been helped by the various lumbar-support products out on the market. These are sometimes called prenatal cradles, and are essentially girdle-like contraptions that offer support, and they are available at some maternity stores. I have never used one, so I can't vouch for them personally.

In addition to lower back pain, some pregnant women also experience *upper* back pain, which is caused by the weight of newly huge breasts, and can be helped considerably by going out and treating yourself to a really good, supportive bra. Now is not the time for something filmy and sheer; stick with heavy-duty, spandex material throughout.

• **Sciatica.** Sometimes, as the fetus grows, its weight falls on the sciatic nerve, sending a shooting pain along the buttocks and down the legs. Massage can help, as can exercise and bed rest. The good news is that sciatica doesn't persist, but usually comes and goes with no predictable regularity.

• **Dizziness and fainting.** Dizziness is a fairly common sensation during the second trimester, and is most likely caused by nothing more than the fact that your blood pressure has dropped, and that you're prone to a sudden drop when you change position quickly, as when you jump out of bed. Try to make your movements slower and more deliberate.

Another common scenario is one in which you'll be standing around, doing nothing out of the ordinary—waiting in line at the supermarket or the bank—when suddenly the room starts to spin. Standing still allows the blood to pool in the lower half of the body, so the brain isn't getting the circulation it needs. If you feel the room start to spin, or feel as though you might even faint, common sense dictates that you should lie down with your feet elevated. Or else, as you've probably heard recommended for garden-variety dizziness as well, sit with your head between your knees. Be sure to tell your doctor about any such episodes; while they're not life-threatening, this is the kind of information we like to track.

• **Hemorrhoids.** It's the rare pregnant woman who hasn't experienced at least a mild form of hemorrhoids, a condition that up until pregnancy seemed to be something remote and embarrassing, relegated to subway ads. What hemorrhoids are, actually, are varicose veins located in your rectum. Just as you might have experienced varicosities of the leg or labia, the veins of your rectum can also swell up during this time. Among the non-pregnant population, overweight people tend to get hemorrhoids most, as do people who are constipated and strain a lot on the toilet. But hemorrhoids are common in pregnancy, and can often linger well past delivery. Here are a few ways to avoid and/or manage them:

1. *Drink plenty of fluids,* even more than the current oceanic amount you're drinking. This will help avoid constipation.

2. *If you are constipated, ask your doctor whether you can take Metamucil or some other form of fiber, or be given a stool softener.*

3. *Don't strain when you're on the toilet.*

4. *Take warm baths.* Sitz baths—little plastic tubs you can sit in—are sold in drug stores, and many women find them useful and soothing once hemorrhoids have formed.

5. *Use Tucks pads.* You can even refrigerate them for a cooling relief.

6. *Use over-the-counter hemorrhoid creams or suppositories if your doctor gives you the okay.* One combination that I personally found to work was a standard hemorrhoid cream such as Preparation H used in conjunction with an anesthetic cream called Tronothane, which is made of one percent pramoxine hydrochloride.

• **Incontinence.** Somewhere around the 20-week mark, you may notice that you don't exert the usual control over your bladder. Especially during coughs or sneezes, you may find yourself involuntarily losing small spurts of urine. Sometimes the movement of the fetus can create a "spasm" of the bladder, resulting in a brief release of urine. This loss of bladder control is completely normal, certainly not shameful, and no cause for concern.

Technically, incontinence is a complete loss of bladder control, which is not what we're talking about here. But for

most women, even occasional—or what we call episodic—
incontinence is a new experience. Usually it occurs during
valsalvas—any movements that increase abdominal pressures, including (in addition to those I mentioned in the
preceding paragraph) bowel movements and laughter. In
the later stages of pregnancy, it's not uncommon for some
women to confuse an episode of incontinence with their
water breaking. (Never try to affect your urinary output by
drinking less water. This can lead to dehydration problems
for yourself and the fetus.)

• **Bleeding.** I've received many telephone calls in the middle of the workday or late at night from women in the second trimester who have suddenly begun bleeding. This is a
frightening experience for them, and of course their immediate thought is that they're having a miscarriage. But I'm
not so quick to jump to that conclusion. One of the first
questions I ask is whether they've had intercourse recently.
Sometimes the capillaries in the vagina can be injured, and
because the vulva are so engorged, there can be an impressive amount of blood released. This isn't dangerous, and
will usually resolve itself.

Another thought I might have is whether the bleeding
could be from hemorrhoids. When a woman wipes herself
with toilet paper and sees blood, she may naturally assume
the blood is vaginal, when in fact it's rectal.

Yet another condition that causes bleeding is a cervical
polyp, which may have been around for a long time but has
only now become visible because of the changes in the
cervix that take place during pregnancy. A cervical polyp is a
benign growth on the cervix, which is prone to inflammation and bleeding. If this is the case, then I'll keep the
patient on pelvic rest. I won't try to remove the polyp during

pregnancy, because of the risk of excessive bleeding, but will remove it during delivery or else wait until after delivery.

If a woman starts bleeding and she has placenta previa (a condition I described on page 87, in which the placenta is overlying the cervix, blocking the exit of the uterus), I have to determine whether she's gone into premature labor. If so, I'll put her on bed rest and try to stop any contractions with drugs called tocolytics that are specifically designed for that purpose (for more on this subject, see page 123). Later in the pregnancy, we'll repeat the sonogram to see if the placenta has moved out of the way, and in nearly all cases, it does. Normally, as the uterus grows upward, so does the placenta, lifting it away from the cervix and clearing the birth canal. If not, though, we make plans for a cesarean section at term. We would also plan a C-section if the patient has undergone previous fibroid surgery, or currently has a fibroid blocking the birth canal, a condition (similar to placenta previa) called tumor previa.

Of course, very, very rarely, a woman does lose a pregnancy in the second trimester, and bleeding is in fact the start of a miscarriage or preterm delivery (see also page 33). Like those in the first trimester, second-trimester miscarriages can be the result of a genetic abnormality in the fetus, but they also might signal a serious problem with the mother or her uterus—an intrauterine infection, perhaps, or an abnormal size or shape of the uterus (congenital uterine malformation) that might be the result of her mother's use of DES (diethylstilbestrol), a drug that used to be given to women to help prevent miscarriage and other pregnancy-related disorders, and which was later found to cause medical problems—cancer and malformations—in some of the daughters of these women.

A rare condition called incompetent cervix—a cervix that opens prematurely without contractions—also can be the cause of a second-trimester miscarriage, if unrecognized and untreated. An obstetrician might consider this diagnosis if a woman has a history of any of the following: a previous second-trimester loss; previous cone biopsy of the cervix; previous trauma to the cervix; DES exposure. If caught in time, though, a miscarriage might be prevented through a procedure called cerclage, in which the cervix is stitched closed, ideally until term.

Sometimes, however, a miscarriage begins, and nothing can be done to stop it. Later, we'll try to determine the cause of the miscarriage, and to see whether it can be avoided in future pregnancies. In my practice, I remember each and every second-trimester miscarriage, partly because they're so unusual, and partly because they're so emotionally wrenching.

RISK OF PREMATURITY

Premature delivery is something that all obstetricians work to avoid, and something that I was quite afraid of myself when I was pregnant. I knew that twins have a higher rate of prematurity, and I really wanted to keep the babies inside me as long as I could, having seen all too well what can happen when a baby is born too early.

The idea of premature delivery worries doctors so much because while many of these early babies ultimately thrive, others do not. The outcome depends on factors such as exactly how premature the baby is, how much the baby weighs, and how developed his or her lungs are at the time of birth. Preemies have a potential for any number of problems, and labor and delivery are believed to be quite diffi-cult for them, even traumatic. Babies who are born very prematurely (usually that means before 32 weeks) can develop intracranial bleeding and neurological abnormali-ties. Also, preemies are more prone to respiratory diseases even after their lungs mature.

I've seen babies who were born at 24 to 26 weeks, and in my experience these are the hardest cases to deal with. There is indeed viability, but sometimes in such instances we see the glaring difference between intact survival and mere sur-vival. Some very early preemies are ultimately neurologically normal, but many suffer long-term complications.

All of which brings me to my most emphatic point: If there is some inkling that a baby is going to arrive early—indicated either by the onset of premature labor or a past premature delivery—there are specific actions that can be taken to improve the outcome. One of the most powerful weapons in the obstetrician's arsenal is to give a patient drugs known as antenatal steroids. Steroids have been shown to speed up fetal lung maturity. Steroids don't seem to do any harm, and in fact those babies whose mothers were treated with steroids experience a lower rate of respi-ratory distress. I was disturbed to come across a recent study reporting that only about 20 percent of patients at risk for delivering prematurely are receiving steroids. If you have a risk factor for premature delivery, I strongly urge you to talk to your doctor about the possibility of receiving steroids.

Candidates for antenatal steroids include women who:

1. *Have a history of preterm labor*

2. *Are having multiple births*

3. *Have had cervical trauma or surgery on the cervix*

4. *Are currently experiencing preterm labor.*

When I started having premature contractions at 31 weeks, my doctor administered antenatal steroids, and I'm convinced that this is what helped my twins a week and a half later. Samantha weighed 4 lbs. 7 oz., and Zachary weighed 3 lbs. 13 oz., and they both stayed in the special care nursery for 13 days, because they had problems associated with their small size. Small babies have trouble maintaining their temperature and need to be in incubators, and they often have feeding problems. My kids were small but healthy; their lungs were in good shape and neither one required any oxygen. I think steroids played a significant role in preventing pulmonary problems.

As I mentioned earlier, another option for women at risk for premature delivery are drugs called tocolytics, which are designed to stave off early contractions. These are widely used, though not without temporary side effects. Terbutaline causes jitteriness, a racing heart, and shortness of breath. Magnesium sulfate, which is administered intravenously in the hospital, can cause sedation, hot flushing, and headaches.

Also widely prescribed is plain old bed rest, although this option remains somewhat controversial because no one can measure its effectiveness in quantitative terms. Cost-benefit analysis, for instance, hasn't found any statistical support for bed rest, but as I mentioned earlier regarding this subject, I'm less interested in an economist's estimate of what lost work time might be costing society than I am in the well-being of the patient in my office.

Gravity does have an effect on the cervix; some uterine

activity levels have been linked to the patient's overall physical activity. These are the factors that weigh most heavily for me. Women get upset when I order them to drop everything and lie down (preferably leaning toward the left, to improve blood flow to the uterus), sometimes for weeks or even months. They bargain with me, trying to get me to soften my orders. Generally, these are the same women who earlier in pregnancy tried to convince me to let them go snowmobiling, etc. It's as though they still don't seem to understand how seriously I take their pregnancies, and how seriously they should, too.

I had one patient, herself a doctor, whom I put on bed rest at 30 weeks. She balked, telling me how busy her own practice was, and how her patients were going to go insane and die without her. I answered that I really wanted her to reach 34 weeks without delivering, and that she'd simply have to find someone to cover her practice in the interim. So she did, muttering all the while. Now she's at 39 weeks, home free, and of course she thinks I was foolish to put her on bed rest in the first place. But who's to say whether she would have done as well as she did if she had run around treating her own patients and leading her usual non-stop, high-wire, active life?

I'd rather err on the side of caution than endanger a pregnancy. I don't want to be kicking myself after the fact, wondering why I gave in and let some high-powered executive keep working after she pleaded with me. So, my advice to you is: *Don't plead with your doctor.*

If your doctor's gut instinct is to confine you to bed, well, then . . . stay in that bed. The Superwoman complex can lead to problems. Doctors are human, and it's just possible that you could actually be persuasive enough to talk your doctor into changing his or her mind and allowing you to be up and about more than is good for you. Sometimes, a patient can be a tough negotiator: What if she took a car service to the office? What if she set up an office at home?

Sometimes she gets her way and it all goes fine—no board meetings are missed, no shareholders are angry—and the child is born looking ready for a photo shoot for Baby Gap.

But other times things don't go as well as we'd hoped. If you are the type of person who snapped to attention when I mentioned the term "Superwoman," then listen closely: In my opinion, the true Superwoman has enough wisdom to follow orders when a doctor says something might be brewing. Every day that we can "buy" toward reaching full term saves two days that your baby would have spent in the intensive care unit. And if you think bed rest is tough, compared to visiting your baby in intensive care, it's a piece of cake.

the
third
trimester

Chapter Seven
Are We There Yet?

- Aches and Pains
- Decreased Fetal Movement and Growth Concerns
- Hypertension and Preeclampsia
- Final Tests
- Preparing for Delivery

What a difference a trimester makes. One week a pregnant woman can be feeling wonderful—filled with a sense of well-being and freed of both nausea and fatigue—and then the next week, the third trimester hits. Now the pregnancy begins to take a profound physical toll. The presence of extra weight tends to induce musculoskeletal pain. The fatigue returns, too, often with a vengeance. It's as though the second trimester were merely a reprieve, a furlough, and now it's time to return to the serious work of creating another human life.

ACHES AND PAINS

In my experience, while women suffer from a variety of physical complaints during the third trimester, the symptoms are easier for them to understand than they had been during the first trimester. Back then, all the nausea, exhaustion, and those peculiar bodily sensations seemed excessive, given that the "baby" was so tiny and abstract. The changes of the first trimester take place on a subtler chemical and hormonal level, but those of the third involve the much more obvious strains of carrying around both extra weight and extra fluid.

At around 32 weeks, women may find that back pain peaks. This is the point at which pain is also felt intensely in the hips, due to the continued relaxation of pelvic ligaments in preparation for the passage of a baby. As the baby's head settles into the pelvis, it creates a wedge that forces the mother's bones and ligaments to be pushed outward laterally. The sacroiliac joint in the lower back gets a real clobbering now from the extra cargo of pregnancy, and many women experience chronic back problems that last for months to come.

One of the most common places that pain tends to collect at this point is around the front of the body, directly under the ribs on the right-hand side. There's no real explanation for this; it just seems, anatomically, to be a choice place for a baby's body parts to settle, and as a result women often experience tenderness in that particular region. The entire area surrounding the uterus gets very sore, too. (In my own third trimester, I felt as though I had been punched in that spot repeatedly.) The vagina itself may feel sore from further engorgement of the tissues.

Patients often tell me of a sensation of vaginal pressure, even though the baby's head is nowhere near; it's merely the increase in blood volume and fluid that creates this often unpleasant feeling.

The accumulation of fluid can cause problems elsewhere in the body as well, particularly in the hands and feet. In the hands, pregnant women often experience carpal tunnel syndrome, an ailment that involves the tendinous sheath that wraps around the wrist below the skin. As the sheath expands with water it turns into a kind of sponge, and the buildup of fluid sometimes compresses the underlying nerves. Carpal tunnel syndrome primarily affects fingers 2 through 4—the index finger, middle finger, and ring finger—causing painful stiffness that usually gets worse as the day progresses. Generally speaking, this is not a serious condition, and just about 99.9 percent of cases will resolve after delivery. I try to tell women to hang on, that they will feel better soon enough. But if the stiffness and pain are extremely severe and debilitating, I will recommend a wrist splint that can be worn at night.

Changes in the feet can be equally intense, and my patients often complain of swelling or burning on the soles. I always take a look at, and a quick feel of, a woman's ankles at office visits, to see if there's excessive water retention there, which could possibly be related to a developing case of preeclampsia, a serious condition I will discuss later in this chapter. I personally felt an intense "burn" on the bottoms of my feet, and I would often come home from work and rub my bare, scorched, itchy feet on the carpet like a dog.

One other side effect of all this excess fluid is rare but worth a mention. Sometimes the fluid collects within the lens of the eye, and women can find themselves in need of glasses with a new prescription for the final stages of the pregnancy.

At night, when sleep takes over, women are susceptible to another type of problem: leg cramps. There's no definitive consensus as to what causes them, which makes them more difficult to treat than other symptoms. There are lots of theories floating around, having to do with calcium and magnesium levels, but no one really knows the answer. If you wake up in the night with a painful leg cramp, the best way to relieve the pain is to stretch out the leg and flex the foot, the way you might treat a charley horse.

On top of all these problems, the breasts are larger than ever and extremely cumbersome, and some women develop stretch marks (striae) there and elsewhere, especially in the hips. Stretch marks, which are an overdistension of the skin, are caused by the breakdown of the normal network of collagen fibers. There's definitely a genetic component to stretch marks; women whose mothers don't have stretch marks on their bodies tend to have fewer themselves. It's not that there's an actual gene for stretch marks, but parents do pass a certain "skin integrity" on to their children. When women tell me they hate their stretch marks and will never want to wear a bikini again, I am sympathetic. The fact is, the marks never completely go away, although they certainly fade. Some dermatologists claim to have been getting good results with vitamin E cream and, more recently, Retin-A cream (which should *never* be used during pregnancy, only in its aftermath). If stretch marks are particularly severe and a woman is unhappy about them, I'll suggest she see a dermatologist once the baby is born. In the meantime, I'm sorry to say that there is nothing that can be done to prevent them. Nobody can change the way their skin reacts to being stretched so severely.

For some women, an intensely itchy abdomen is yet one more side effect of the skin's stretching. There is another syndrome, whose acronym is PUPPPS (pruritic urticarial papules and plaques of pregnancy), which generally develops in the late third trimester. Treatment consists of anti-itch measures such as Caladryl lotion, Benadryl, or Aveeno baths, which are made of soothing oatmeal flakes. It's important for a woman with PUPPPS not to scratch, because she could inflame the area and cause a skin infection. In severe cases I'll recommend that she wear socks on her hands at night, so she can't tear at her skin in her sleep, and I'll possibly prescribe a cortisone cream. And in *extremely* severe cases, in which the itching is uncontrollable, I will run further tests. Some forms of itching are associated with a liver function abnormality (cholestasis); the bile salts get backed up and deposited in the skin, where they can cause this kind of constant itching. This condition may even call for earlier delivery, since delivery is the only known cure.

Speaking of constant itching, some pregnant women develop various annoying rashes on other areas of their body, such as the arms or legs; again, their obstetricians can prescribe low-dose cortisone creams.

Which brings me to another, unrelated topic: constant urinating. This is a common complaint shared by most of my patients. As I mentioned earlier, it tends to be a problem early in the pregnancy, then abates in the middle months, only to return with a vengeance in the third trimester. I know of very few women in the final months of their pregnancy who are able to sleep through the night without having to get up and urinate at least a couple of times.

The baby itself makes its presence known more and more, not only through these indelicate and uncomfortable symptoms, but perhaps also through mini-contractions known as Braxton-Hicks contractions. The uterus, in order to successfully dilate the cervix, has to get the hang of contracting, and Braxton-Hicks are essentially a practice run-through of the real thing. Sometimes women become frightened when they feel these sudden sensations of tightening across the abdomen, worrying that they have gone into premature labor. But I reassure my patients that the presence of Braxton-Hicks contractions does *not* mean that they are going into labor. (I also tell them that the absence of Braxton-Hicks contractions is not worrisome, either. Some women just never experience them.) How to tell the difference? True labor pains, when they eventually start, will occur rhythmically, organizing themselves into a pattern, whereas Braxton-Hicks are disorganized contractions that start and stop at random. Women shouldn't be afraid, but should be impressed by the body's amazing ability to stage a rehearsal for the big event.

Between the variety of aches and pains and preoccupations you are now experiencing, the tranquility of the second trimester may start to feel like a fading dream. It's not only you, the patient, who pays more attention to the medical minutiae of the pregnancy now; your doctor also becomes more focused. Office visits are more frequent, as I mentioned earlier, usually every two to three weeks up until week 36, then, in the last month, once a week. During third-trimester office visits, your obstetrician is specifically concerned with the following details, for reasons that will become clear throughout the rest of this chapter:

• Blood pressure.
• Protein in the urine.

• Weight gain.

• Edema (sudden swelling of the feet, and possibly the hands and face, which warrants an immediate call to your doctor).

DECREASED FETAL MOVEMENT AND GROWTH CONCERNS

Your doctor is also focusing more on your specific perceptions of fetal movement. A true decrease in fetal movement could be the first indication of a worrisome development. I'm very interested in what my patients tell me they're feeling. If a woman calls and says she's worried that her baby hasn't been moving around very much that day, I tell her the following: Have a small meal, then lie on your side and concentrate on fetal movement. If you notice ten movements within a half-hour period, you can feel totally reassured that things are fine, and so can I. But if you don't notice ten movements, then pick up the phone and call me back.

Several factors can affect a woman's ability to discern fetal movement: what she's doing (a more active lifestyle can mask the movements); the position of the fetus (especially if the baby is in the breech position—see page 160); decreased amniotic fluid level. If we're concerned about decreased fetal movement, we'll order a non-stress test, which is a noninvasive way to determine the fetal heart rate pattern (for a full description of an NST, see page 138), and a sonogram, which will measure the volume of amniotic fluid. The fetal movement pattern in some women—those with underlying hypertension, diabetes, or other risk factors for fetal complications—automatically merits special attention, and I'll have those patients assess fetal movement every day.

All babies go through sleep and wake cycles that affect how much and how often they move. Usually when a woman is worried about decreased movement, her fears turn out to be unwarranted. Babies get quiet in there; sometimes this calm, still state is very much akin to settling down for the night.

(As always, if there are any dramatic changes in your baby's movements, you should let your doctor know.)

In addition to fetal movement, the doctor will concentrate on fundal height, assessing the growth of the fetus by determining how high the uterus extends. This is literally a hands-on measurement: The doctor will place his or her hands on your abdomen. Some doctors prefer to use a tape measure. If the fundal height seems to lag behind the expected size for your due date, the doctor will wonder if the discrepancy is due either to the size of the fetus or to the amount of amniotic fluid, and you may be sent for a sonogram to make sure there isn't intrauterine growth retardation (IUGR) or oligohydramnios. The later the sonogram, however, the greater the margin of error in assessing the growth of the fetus. Eventually, by the third trimester, the margin of error is 15 percent—the difference, in some cases, between worrying and not worrying. For better or worse, however, comparing individual results to "normal" growth curves helps determine whether the fetus is growing appropriately. If the growth of the fetus *does* seem to be slowing down, you may be placed on bed rest to increase blood flow and shunt nutrients to the baby. You will be sent for another sonogram to follow fetal growth. In addition, the development of the fetal lungs might be accelerated with steroids in case it becomes necessary to deliver early, in order to get the baby out of what may be becoming an inhospitable environment.

The reason that office visits become so frequent is that this is the time that certain complications, if they're going to develop, may set in. I want to go into detail here about our most common precautions, which include close monitoring for hypertensive disorders as well as a few final tests for anemia, diabetes, and Group B strep.

HYPERTENSION AND PREECLAMPSIA

You probably haven't paid all that much attention to the nurse who takes your blood pressure at every visit, but doctors look at these readings very closely, especially now. Any elevations in the third trimester above the baseline (which was established at your first visit) may signal the development of pregnancy-induced hypertension, also known as PIH.

I think of hypertension as encompassing a broad spectrum, with simple pregnancy-induced hypertension at one end, and preeclampsia and eclampsia at the other. How I decide to treat a woman with PIH depends on a variety of specifics. As is the case with most potential complications, I'm constantly weighing two factors: the health of the mother and the environment of the baby.

Every situation is different, of course, and needs to be treated as an individual case. If a woman develops high blood pressure—meaning either the systolic reading is over 140 (or, alternatively, at least 30 points higher than the baseline established at her first visit), or the diastolic is over 90 (or at least 15 points higher than the baseline)—we have to take into account the gestational age of the fetus. If it's 32 weeks, for instance, and the mother is becoming hypertensive, there's a definite advantage to aggressively treating the mother's blood pressure with medications and bed rest—that is, to being conservative and keeping a close watch—as opposed to simply delivering the baby so early. (If the baby were 37 weeks, however, I would induce labor at that point and feel relieved that I'd gotten the baby out of what might well have been deteriorating uterine conditions.) What I mean by "keeping a close watch" is conducting safe, noninvasive monitoring such as a non-stress test (NST), which gives us some insight into the overall status of the fetus as well as an idea of how efficiently the placenta is delivering oxygen and nutrients.

The placenta provides the sole communication between the mother and the fetus. The umbilical cord winds from the fetus to the inside wall of the placenta, and inside the umbilical cord run the blood vessels that exchange nutrients and oxygen with the mother's blood supply. Any condition that affects the ability of the placenta to provide for the fetus is therefore worth monitoring closely.

A non-stress test usually takes place in the doctor's office, although some doctors who don't have the equipment available send the woman to the hospital as an outpatient. Before an NST, a nurse attaches two monitors to a woman's abdomen, using conducting gel and a wide elastic belt to hold the monitors in place. Then she will have the woman lie back on the examining table while the machine, called a fetal monitor, records the fetus's heartbeat as well as any fetal movements and uterine contractions on a scroll of paper. (If you've had an EKG, the experience will be familiar.) There's a volume control on the machine, and usually the nurse or doctor will leave the volume up so that the fetus's heartbeat can be heard thumping valiantly away. Basically, the non-stress test checks to make sure that the baby is responding properly *in utero*. Whenever a woman feels her baby move, the baby's heart rate usually accelerates—the same way, when you perform some physical activity, your own heartbeat speeds up.

During an NST, a woman will be told to lie on a table and remain hooked up to the monitor until a "reactive tracing" is obtained, which means until the doctor feels reassured by the pattern on the printout. Theoretically, this takes only 20 minutes to accomplish, but in reality I find that it can take longer. The baby has its own sleep and wake cycles, and what might seem, initially, to be a reading indicative of a non-reactive baby, may prove to be indicative of nothing more than a baby that's fast asleep. If you are given an NST and it takes more than 20 minutes to achieve a reactive tracing, I wouldn't jump to the conclusion that something is wrong. I sometimes give my patients a cup of orange juice or a few ice chips to stimulate the baby. (The non-stress test, by the way, like all noninvasive testing, is painless.)

If the test shows something ominous or simply doesn't give me enough reassurance—little variability, or a lack of accelerations, or the presence of decelerations—I might want to get more information. One option would be to send a patient out for a stress (as opposed to non-stress) test, commonly called an Oxytocin Challenge Test (OCT). The test is done at the hospital, with the woman attached to a continuous fetal monitor. We administer a low dose of oxytocin by infusion to stimulate uterine contractions (known by its brand name, Pitocin). An adequate test is when she experiences three mild contractions within a ten-minute period. (For more on Pitocin, see page 174). These contractions "stress" the baby, enabling us to see, based on the fetal heart tracing, how the baby responds: Does the heart rate accelerate, stay the same, or does it decelerate? Essentially, we get some idea of how the baby would handle true, full-blown labor—and, based on this, we can decide whether the pregnancy should be allowed to continue, or whether we need to deliver ahead of schedule.

Another tool we have for assessing fetal health is the sonogram, which can estimate fetal growth and the level of amniotic fluid, both of which are associated with blood flow to the baby. If a woman has developed pregnancy-specific complications such as high blood pressure or diabetes, or there's evidence that the fetus isn't growing appropriately, her doctor may recommend a more detailed sonogram called a biophysical profile (BPP). This sonogram assesses the following:

- Fetal movement
- Fetal tone
- Fetal breathing
- Amniotic fluid volume.

The first three items on this list start to falter when a baby is stressed. If these readings are found to be abnormal, my scale tends to tip in favor of getting the baby out—provided, of course, that the mother is stable. The fact is, even though I'm worried about both patients, the mother's well-being has to come before her baby's.

If a woman whose blood pressure has risen into the hypertensive range also starts spilling protein into her urine (determined by the dipstick test done at each visit) and developing edema in her hands and face, then she has moved from a diagnosis of PIH into preeclampsia.

Preeclampsia, which in the past was called toxemia, usually presents three major symptoms: hypertension, edema (swelling), and protein in the urine. It's a serious condition that compromises the welfare of both mother and fetus. It can also turn into a life-threatening condition called eclampsia, which is characterized by seizures and can lead to coma. Eclampsia is a true medical emergency; while obviously dangerous to the mother, it also can compromise the blood flow to the baby.

Most preeclampsia, however, if diagnosed properly, doesn't develop into eclampsia. It is either kept under control through antiseizure medication such as magnesium sulfate, or is resolved by delivering the baby. Once the baby is out, the mother's blood pressure generally lowers dramatically within the next 24 to 48 hours.

Nobody knows for sure what causes preeclampsia. It's almost as though some women are allergic to being pregnant, and their bodies simply treat the placenta as a foreign agent that has no business being there. An analogous situation occurs when you get a grain of sand in your eye, and your eye floods with tears. The body of a preeclamptic woman seems to recognize what's not part of itself and demands its expulsion. Most women's bodies, however, treat the baby as a natural extension of the mother, and have no problem with its presence on board.

If you are one of those women whose blood pressure suddenly shoots up, you should know that while PIH and preeclampsia are very serious and need to be followed closely and treated, your doctor has definitely seen this before, and will see it again. (Sometimes, a woman who has experienced preeclampsia in one pregnancy may be prescribed extra calcium supplements or even baby aspirin in the next pregnancy, since some recent studies have shown this might reduce the likelihood of the condition recurring.) Although PIH can arrive as early as 20 weeks, it is much more likely to develop in the third trimester. Sometimes we see it as early as six weeks before term, and sometimes we don't diagnose it until the patient is in labor.

If your blood pressure is elevated and you're still several weeks from term, your doctor will probably first order bed rest. One of the many things I worry about even in a borderline PIH patient is impaired blood flow to the baby. I always tell these patients that they have no choice but to take it easy, and I'm serious. If a woman has extremely high blood pressure, now is the time for her to drop everything, to quit her job, to call off all her engagements, and to stay at home and rest. I recommend that she lie in bed on her left side, which helps favor blood flow toward the uterus.

Preeclampsia received a little extra attention a few years ago, when the television show "E.R." ran an episode that featured a woman in labor who came to the emergency room because the labor floor was overbooked, and in the middle of her labor developed preeclampsia, then eclampsia, and finally died. The show was very disturbing to most of my pregnant patients who watched it. The day after the show aired, my office telephone was ringing off the hook. "I'm afraid I'm going to die," one woman said, her voice still trembling. "I'm just so scared to go through delivery now."

Women tend to be scared enough of delivery to begin with, without having a television show escalate their fears. As I told my patients at the time, the fallacy of the episode lay in the fact that, in a major metropolitan hospital with an obstetrics department, there is no way that a pregnant woman would remain in the emergency room. If platelet numbers drop or there are liver or kidney function abnormalities, this is evidence of a life-threatening problem, and a pregnant woman in that condition would be rushed like lightning to the labor floor. My point here is that, regardless of how overcrowded your labor floor may be, and regardless of what kinds of medical complications may arise in your pregnancy, it's *extremely, extremely* rare for a woman to be allowed to get so critically ill in pregnancy that she dies. One of the reasons for the low maternal mortality rate in the United States is that doctors who monitor a patient with complications know they may very well induce labor early, if need be. If a woman has preeclampsia, I'm generally looking for a reason to get her delivered. The stability of the situation can change from day to day, so I'm constantly reassessing the risks and benefits of delivery.

If you have preeclampsia and your doctor orders you to stay home from work, I strongly urge you not to argue. Go home, lie on your left side, and stay there. I can't tell you how many times I've had patients who haven't followed orders, women who are so zealous that they sneak into their office for a few hours of work. It's as though these women think I'm ordering them to stay home just to be mean. They chafe at my authority and want to defy me, as though they're rebellious teenagers and I'm their mom. If your blood pressure is up and your doctor tells you to take it easy, this is sound medical advice that needs to be followed.

Sometimes either before or during delivery, I give women with preeclampsia a rather effective but unpleasant drug called magnesium sulfate, known as mag sulfate for short. It protects against the seizures of eclampsia, but unfortunately it also makes patients flushed, hot, and headachy. Women on mag sulfate aren't allowed to get out of bed even to go to the bathroom, and must remain on the drug for at least 24 hours after delivery. This is often frustrating for women who have just given birth, because they typically aren't allowed to "room in" with their newborns. (Some hospitals don't allow women to breast-feed until the mag is out of their system, which can also be upsetting.) They're often put on total bed rest, with a Foley catheter to drain their urine and monitor their urine output each hour. These patients can feel extremely drugged and out of it, as well as a bit like a pincushion, with blood being drawn from them every six hours. But mag sulfate dramatically lowers the chance of a seizure, and it remains one of the most powerful ways we have of keeping a serious medical condition from becoming life-threatening to both mother and baby.

FINAL TESTS

As we enter the home stretch, we'll also be guarding closely against three other potential complications: diabetes, anemia, and Group B strep. None of these is likely to affect you, but then, none is so uncommon that it's not worth mentioning.

• **Diabetes.** In my practice, we perform tests for diabetes twice: a glucose screen at 16 weeks (at the time of the AFP), in order to rule out the occasional case of previously unrecognized pre-gestational diabetes, and once again between 28 and 30 weeks. The hormones of pregnancy don't usually cause gestational diabetes until well into the second or even the third trimester, and then only in 3 to 5 percent of pregnant women.

We don't rely on risk factors alone to determine whether you're likely to develop gestational diabetes, although they do count for something. Risk factors include:

1. *Obesity.*

2. *Maternal age over 30.*

3. *A family history of diabetes.*

4. *Excessive weight gain during pregnancy.*

These are all useful as signs, but it's not as though I don't offer the screen to women who are 22 and as skinny as Kate Moss. I have everyone screened. Gestational diabetes is one of the easier problems in pregnancy to regulate, and when brought under control the risks to mother and baby are reduced to the level of a nondiabetic's.

The glucose screen (given at 28 to 30 weeks) is a nonfasting test in which you have to drink half a bottle of some very sweet glucose liquid, usually either orange- or cola-flavored, 60 minutes prior to having your blood drawn. The label on the bottle warns about all kinds of side effects that you might feel after drinking it, such as dizziness, nausea, and bloating. I have to say that even though I have rarely known a patient to have an adverse reaction to this stuff, I was nervous myself when it came time for me to drink it. I had always warned women that the drink wouldn't taste good, but to my surprise, I found that I actually liked the taste. It was not unlike a syrupy, old-fashioned fountain soda. It's also more palatable when cold, or poured over ice. Fifty grams of glucose is a lot of sweet stuff to ingest, but if you looked at the side of a box of sweetened breakfast cereal, you'd probably find 50 grams of glucose per serving, and no warnings whatsoever about dizziness, nausea, or bloating. The glucose screen is no big deal. But untreated diabetes *is* a big deal, so it's important that you get tested.

A small percentage of women do have an elevated screen, and as a result I have them take a fasting, three-hour, entire-bottle glucose tolerance test. The risks associated with diabetes in pregnancy are significant: Some women deliver macrosomic babies, which, as I've mentioned, means babies that weigh over eight pounds, thirteen ounces, and tend to have a different distribution of body fat, which can make delivery more difficult and even dangerous. Also, there is a higher mortality rate *in utero*, as well as increased amniotic fluid, which makes the uterus larger and leads to a greater risk of preterm labor.

A woman with gestational diabetes can control the condition by modifying her diet. Basically, the recommended diet is one that is high in protein and calories and low in carbohydrates. She'll be told to dramatically cut down on her intake of carbohydrates, such as bread and bagels. (One bagel, by the way, equals *five* slices of bread; I haven't eaten a bagel since I heard that.) A diabetic will instead eat more cheese, eggs, lean meats, and peanut butter (which is a popular favorite). Fruit juices aren't allowed.

She also has to monitor her blood sugar throughout the day, using what are called "finger-sticks." The patient is given a disposable needle, with which she pricks her finger. A small drop of blood is placed on a test strip and a compact machine called a home glucose monitor analyzes that specimen. She checks her blood sugar first thing in the morning (called a fasting specimen), and then one hour after a meal (called a postprandial specimen). Diabetic women in my practice are counseled about dietary changes. If you are found to have gestational diabetes and your doctor gives you a diet to follow, you might ask if there is a nurse or nutritionist affiliated with the practice who can help you with the significant adjustments you'll need to make.

Medically speaking, gestational diabetes is an inability to metabolize carbohydrates appropriately. As I've said, most women bring the condition under control simply with dietary changes, though occasionally a patient will be unable to control the diabetes, and will need to take insulin. We're very strict about monitoring gestational diabetes, because we've got not one but two patients to worry about. Tight control ensures a much better outcome. If you're a gestational diabetic, try to view the situation this way: The whole thing is a royal pain in the neck and a big obligation, but if you do what you're told you will very likely reduce your risks dramatically.

I always screen a gestational diabetic again six weeks after her baby is born, because if she's had diabetes in pregnancy, she's at a much greater risk for adult-onset diabetes. At six weeks postpartum, the vast majority of gestational diabetes cases will have cleared, though women diagnosed with diabetes during one pregnancy do tend to develop diabetes during subsequent pregnancies, and about half these women will develop it in middle age.

I've had patients come to me and complain that they don't want to undergo the glucose screen, and that during their last pregnancy, when they lived outside of New York, their doctors never made them take the test. I'm not persuaded by these complaints and arguments. I believe you should take the test at least once during your pregnancy, and that if for some reason your doctor doesn't automatically order it (and some doctors don't), you should ask to have it done.

Women who enter pregnancy already diabetic present an entirely different sort of situation. They're already sophisticated about diet changes and insulin and finger-sticks. Usually, though, they're highly nervous about being pregnant, and so are their partners. They've all heard horror stories about bad things happening to the babies of serious diabetics, and the risks, *if* the preexisting diabetes is left uncontrolled, are indeed real: an increased rate of congenital malformations such as anencephaly, spina bifida, and cardiac anomalies. But that's a big—and, in my experience, old and outdated—"if."

I've delivered the babies of several such women, and every outcome has been good. Competent doctors know how to manage diabetic women in pregnancy these days, and most diabetic patients who have their condition under control will do well. With true diabetics, I'll switch their oral medications to injections of insulin, order more frequent ultrasounds to assess the growth of the fetus, and follow with non-stress tests in the third trimester. These days, congenital abnormalities are usually the result of poor glucose control prior to the eighth week of gestation (yet another good reason to schedule that first appointment as early as possible).

• **Anemia.** I routinely check a patient for anemia as part of the basic blood test the first time she comes to see me, but most women are not anemic at that time. Sometimes, though, anemia develops later on. Because of this, I screen for it again at 28 weeks, when the requirements of pregnancy can begin seriously depleting a woman's iron supply.

Severe anemia leaves a woman feeling exhausted and looking quite pale. Sometimes she might be breathless, have heart palpitations, or even pass out. Milder forms of anemia might have no symptoms whatsoever, but can put a woman at risk for severe anemia postpartum. Prenatal vitamins do contain some iron, but if a woman is found to be even mildly anemic I'll also prescribe an iron supplement. This enables a woman to "tank up" prior to delivery, a time we know she'll lose some blood. If I've helped her restore her depleted iron, I feel reassured that she's starting motherhood in optimal condition. She may also want to fortify her diet with extra iron-rich foods, such as red meat, liver, spinach, and dried fruits.

At 28 weeks I perform a complete blood count that looks for possible platelet disorders, which is something I would need to know about before delivery. The platelet test lets us see if there's a problem with clotting; if a woman does have a coagulation disorder, an anesthesiologist might hesitate to put a needle in her back for an epidural. There is a small chance that the fetus will also have a low platelet count, and a vaginal delivery would be too traumatic. So if a test result comes back showing a low platelet count, I will send the woman for a more complete workup. Usually, the disorder turns out to be a benign condition, the patient will be allowed to receive an epidural, and the baby can be delivered vaginally. But as with so many other situations in pregnancy, we need to make sure.

• **Group B Streptococcus.** This is an infection caused by bacteria in the vagina that can be passed on to the baby during delivery. It's not a sexually transmitted infection; instead, it's simply a bacteria that might be naturally found in the vagina of many healthy women, causing them no ill effects. The problem with Group B strep is that it can be passed on to the baby during delivery, and this could be a serious problem for the baby, causing blood infection, fever, or meningitis. Most carriers deliver babies who are *not* infected, but if they are, the results can be devastating. Some practices routinely screen all women at 36 weeks; some others do not screen but treat those who present risk factors, which include:

1. *A previous baby with Group B strep infection.*

2. *Any Group B strep urine infections during the pregnancy.*

3. *Imminent delivery before 37 weeks.*

4. *Ruptured membranes without imminent delivery.*

5. *Fever in labor.*

If a patient tests positive for Group B strep, she'll be treated with antibiotics. You may want to bring up the topic of Group B strep with your doctor to find out where he or she stands with regard to testing.

PREPARING FOR DELIVERY

At this point in a pregnancy, the day of delivery is no longer a vague mirage far off in the distance; now it's approaching rapidly, and seems like more of a reality than it ever did during earlier months. I need to make sure that my patient is in optimized physical shape, and that there are no medical surprises that we will find ourselves confronted with in the labor room.

The patient needs to learn some of the basics of labor and delivery in a relaxed setting, which can best be accomplished by taking a childbirth class. Much of the information is available in videotapes or books, of course, but they're no substitute for a face-to-face question-and-answer session.

Not only are there a number of types of childbirth classes available these days, but they also follow a number of different formats. In the past, women and their partners predictably sat in a circle in a room in a hospital or clinic once a week for six weeks, watching footage of labor and passing around an actual set of forceps. Now couples can even go to a luxury hotel for a weekend crash course.

Which is not to say I think you should; such gimmicky arrangements are likely to be just that: gimmicks. I don't happen to think childbirth classes are essential, but I do think they're enormously helpful for first-time mothers as well as their doctors. Selfishly, perhaps, I feel that some of the onus is taken off the obstetrician if, during a delivery, he or she doesn't have to walk a totally uninformed patient through every detail of what's likely to happen. These classes are also beneficial for couples, especially those expecting for the first time; the classes get them in the habit of thinking of themselves as a parental team, and they're an effective way of involving the father.

Back when all women were encouraged to labor without any anesthesia, these classes were primarily about pain management. There still is a pain-management aspect to most of them, but in a larger sense I think what the classes do best is provide you with a glimpse of what this profound and often unpredictable day or night will really be like.

Childbirth classes are usually offered to women from about the 28th week on; ideally you'd take a class at about 32 weeks. In our practice, we have a nurse from the labor floor give classes in our offices at night. She's someone we work with at the hospital, and because of this she can answer our patients' specific questions about the way babies are delivered in our practice and at our hospital. If your obstetrician has a similar setup, and you can arrange to take classes from a labor nurse affiliated with the hospital where your doctor delivers, I think that's an excellent idea. If this kind of setup isn't available, then be sure to take notes during the class and bring a list of questions to your doctor.

What are casually known as "Lamaze" classes these days aren't usually classes specializing in the Lamaze method so much as general childbirth education classes, which give women and their partners a broad overview of everything from anesthesia to infant care. Sometimes short films are shown that depict women in labor, or women undergoing cesarean sections. Most classes offer a tour of a hospital labor suite, so if you can't take a class through your doctor's office, it might be helpful to take one through the hospital where you will deliver. People tend to be more frightened of scenes they can't really imagine than scenes they can; actually seeing where your baby will be born takes a chunk of mystery (and, along with it, fear) out of the experience.

Some women elect to take classes in what is known as the Bradley Method, which aims for totally drug-free, non-interventional deliveries; women are taught to concentrate on breathing, are discouraged from asking for epidurals, and are taught that episiotomies are to be avoided at all costs. I tend to have a hard time with those patients; the philosophy of the Bradley Method is so different from my own perspective. If a patient were a hardcore Bradleyite, she might be very mistrustful of some of the technology I may need to employ during delivery. She might not, for instance, want a fetal monitor used on her, whereas I feel strongly that a fetal monitor can give me important information. (A fetal monitor is the same piece of equipment as that used in a nonstress test, detailed on page 138.) *Whatever* your feelings about intervention in delivery, I hope you will feel free to discuss them with your doctor now, and not wait to raise them during the zero hour of delivery, when there's rarely enough leisurely time for debate.

Another matter that you should start thinking about now is the choice of a pediatrician. I'm sure the idea of this is pretty strange to you—you haven't even met your baby yet, and already you have to find him or her a doctor. I often give recommendations to patients, but in addition to asking your own obstetrician you can also poll friends who already have children.

Ideally, you'd pick a pediatrician who has privileges at the hospital where you will be delivering; otherwise, he or she won't be allowed to examine the baby after the birth. Instead, one of the attending staff will be selected to perform that initial exam; you'll make an appointment with your own pediatrician for after the baby's been discharged.* The criteria for choosing a pediatrician are not so different from the ones I suggested you use when choosing an obstetrician: Do you feel comfortable with this person? Do you like his or her manner and respect his or her opinions? Is he or she easily reachable by telephone? These questions are particularly relevant now; you'd be surprised how often you may need to call the pediatrician for advice in the early weeks of your baby's life.

Many women and/or their partners, when choosing a pediatrician, go to visit the doctor prior to the birth, to perform what is essentially an "interview" and decide if it's a good match. (Doctors sometimes charge for these appointments, and I don't think that's unfair—after all, they're giving up an appointment's worth of time to you, a stranger.) You should be armed with your own mini-list if you choose to screen a pediatrician, asking any questions you may already have about breast-feeding, vaccinations, circumci-

---

*It may be more important to choose a pediatrician whose office is conveniently located near your home.

sion, as well as the doctor's availability. Be blunt: "*Is it easy to reach you during the day?*" you might well ask. You'll also get a good idea of how a practice works from your experience in the waiting room, if you visit during office hours. Some pediatricians have morning "phone hours," in which they simply sit at their desk and field calls from parents. I think this kind of setup is great, because you don't have to wait all day for a phone call to be returned, especially if you've got a sick baby at home and are anxious.

And then there's the all-important issue of what to take to the hospital when the big moment finally arrives. I hear this question all the time in the third trimester. (Actually, with particularly eager patients, I sometimes hear it in the first trimester.) Patients have become so medically sophisticated these days, discussing sonograms and genetics and placental function, but they often worry that they don't know what to put into their overnight bag. In fact, they don't need to pack anything at all except a change of clothes. As soon as a woman arrives in the labor room she will be given a hospital gown to wear, so she doesn't even have to bring her own nightgown.

The question of whether or not to bring a camera or camcorder often comes up, which to my way of thinking is a personal decision. Many couples arrive at the labor room so well equipped that they look like a film crew for CNN, but other women are horrified at the idea of being photographed in this unglamorous role. Then there are women who want pictures—not of themselves, but of the baby. The only words of wisdom I can offer on this subject is that it would be a shame if a husband or partner experienced the entire birth through a viewfinder. The moment a baby enters the world is always powerful and unforgettable, with or without footage.

Chapter Eight
Ready or Not

- Cervical Exams
- The Baby's Position
- Contractions and Labor
- Ruptured Membranes

Although 37 weeks is the textbook definition of "term," I think of a baby as having achieved maturity at 36 weeks. It's not that I completely disagree with the textbooks; it's simply my belief that babies born from here on in are fully formed and their lungs are almost always fully developed. If a woman goes into labor at this time or needs for some reason to be induced, I feel confident that the delivery will have a positive outcome.

For many pregnant women, the closer they get to delivery the more intensely anxious they become. Obstetricians feel quite differently than patients about the whole matter. Just as I don't view pregnancy as an illness, I also don't view delivery as a dire or emergency medical procedure. While it's true that things sometimes go wrong during deliveries (and every woman seems to be familiar with horror stories—and not just the one from "E.R."), having a baby at the turn of the 21st century—whether vaginally or by cesarean section—is extremely safe. For every 25,000 deliveries in the United States these days, there is only one incident of maternal mortality, and most of these deaths involve serious medical conditions that existed prior to delivery, perhaps even prior to pregnancy.

Although I don't share my patients' increasing anxiety in the final weeks, I do share the accompanying excitement and optimism. After all, delivering babies is the reason obstetricians choose this specialty. Checking urine and blood pressure and listening to a heartbeat are all part of the job, but the real hands-on moment occurs now. There are very few other specialties in which the path of the medical condition is as predictable, or arrives at such a rewarding conclusion. I think it's important for patients to remember that although a delivery is an extremely dramatic experience for the mother, it's not something they should fear. Being admitted to the hospital to have a baby is not like being admitted for a breast biopsy or an emergency appendectomy. It's a natural conclusion to a pregnancy, and yet it seems so daunting because it takes place in a hospital, in the presence of all the high-tech medical machinery that we are lucky enough to have. But I'm getting ahead of myself here. No woman is going to be admitted to the labor floor until she's nearly ready to deliver.

CERVICAL EXAMS

The best way I know to assess readiness is through the cervical exams that are performed in the final weeks of a pregnancy, usually around week 36 or 37, depending upon the doctor's preference. In most cases, a patient will not have been examined internally since her very first visit to my office, simply because there's no useful information to be found in such an exam. If she's not bleeding or cramping, then cervical change is not likely, so why should I subject her to the pointless discomfort of being examined?

What I check for now, after she slowly climbs up onto the table and puts her feet in the stirrups, is the relationship of the baby's head to the "ischial spines," which are the bones that flank the sides of the mother's pelvis, and any change that has taken place in the cervix.

When the baby has "dropped," which you may have also heard referred to as "lightening," he or she is beginning preparations to be born. We don't know for sure what causes a baby to begin the descent, but we do look to this significant clue (or its absence) as an indication of the mother's readiness for labor. When the baby's head is fully engaged, we know with some confidence that the largest part of the baby has entered the pelvis and, barring other complications, can be born vaginally.

Sometimes a pregnant woman definitely knows that her baby has dropped. She'll come into my office and tell me that the placement of the baby feels different to her, and that she's lost that breathless sensation she's been experiencing for weeks—she no longer feels totally stuffed full of baby. But sometimes the baby's descent also causes a woman to feel some new discomfort, which is caused by the baby's head literally pressing down against the pelvis. She might feel this as increased lateral pain in the hips, especially when she's walking, or as groin pain.

I trust my patients when they tell me they've felt a change. But the absence of a felt change isn't particularly meaningful; just as often, women have no idea that the baby has dropped, and they are surprised when I examine them and impart this information. There is no way to know which category you will fall into; over the years I've seen all the permutations. As a rule, we see engagement happening prior to labor only in women who are about to be first-time mothers. With subsequent children, this descent usually occurs during the labor itself.

When the descent has taken place and the widest part of the baby's head has reached the top part of the ischial spines, we call this state "engagement." We measure the extent of the engagement in centimeters, which is also referred to as "station." For instance, you could come in for a cervical exam at 37 weeks and your doctor could find that you're at -5 station, which means your baby has not begun its descent. Later, during delivery itself, the baby moves from 0 station all the way to +5, the latter number being the point at which the head is starting to emerge from the vagina. (This is also known as "crowning," the point at which the head holds the labia apart between contractions.)

These quick measurements are important for a doctor to know. If the head is low, I am reassured that the mother has a good chance of a successful vaginal delivery. If the head is still high up, though, I have to wonder if there's going to be some trouble squeezing through. What I need to assess is whether the baby is, in effect, a square peg in a round hole. You probably won't hear your doctor discuss this in great detail, but station is still one of the things he or she is mentally taking note of during cervical exams.

Another thing your doctor wants to ascertain is whether or not your cervix is starting to "efface," or beginning to get thinner. In order for a woman to deliver vaginally, her cervix needs to eventually thin to the point at which it disappears entirely. We don't know what causes effacement, although we think of it as part of the dissolution of the "cement" that holds together the cervix. As the collagen bundles that make up this "cement" begin to dissolve, the cervix breaks down. Pressure from the baby's head helps this process along, too. By 36 or 37 weeks, significant effacement is rare.

Most pregnant women have a pretty good understanding of the process of cervical dilation that needs to take place during delivery, but they seem to have a less firm grasp on the concept of effacement. And from a doctor's point of view, effacement is a much more meaningful indicator than dilation. In the case of a woman having her first baby, effacement often precedes dilation, and indicates that progress is being made. In my opinion, effacement is the hardest part of the labor process. I'm happy to see some of that work done prior to the onset of true labor. For instance, if a woman's cervix is totally closed but 90 percent effaced, then I feel pretty certain she's going to have a nice, short labor. I've seen it happen time after time. It's always reassuring for a doctor to see effacement occurring early. The absence of effacement makes it harder to assess how things will progress.

Two other factors that I'm considering during a cervical exam are the consistency and the position of the cervix within the vagina. Before any change takes place, the cervix is firm and positioned toward the back of the vagina. This adds to the discomfort of the already dreaded internal exam. With progress, the cervix softens and moves toward the front of the vagina.

But obstetrics is funny. I've often examined a woman in the final weeks of her pregnancy and gotten the sense that the cervix is still firm, uneffaced, and that the head is still high in the pelvis. And yet when labor starts, the baby simply flies through in record time. In my mind, it's always worth giving a woman a chance to deliver vaginally, because I have the safety net of knowing that I'm prepared to resort to a C-section if necessary.

In some practices (though not mine), a doctor may "strip" a woman's membranes during the cervical exam, which means he or she slips a finger between the uterine wall and the sac, which releases prostaglandin, said to stimulate labor.

THE BABY'S POSITION

The garden-variety, head-down position in the uterus, which your baby is likely to assume by the time of its birth, is called the vertex position. This is the preferred position. Because the head is the biggest part of the baby, it makes sense that it ought to be delivered first; after the head is out, mother, baby, and obstetrician are generally home free. But some babies choose not to be vertex, instead stubbornly positioning themselves in a type of breech position, with their buttocks down. This happens more commonly with premature babies, who have more wiggle room in the uterus, and with twins. (It happened to one of my twins, Zachary, who was in a persistent breech position at the end of my pregnancy.)

If, early in the third trimester, your doctor tells you that your baby is currently breech, this isn't anything to worry about. At this time, 15 to 20 percent of all babies will be breech, but by the day they reach term, only 4 to 5 percent will still be in that position; the rest will have flipped themselves around.

If a woman arrives at term—37 weeks—and the baby is still a persistent breech, then it's time to think about attempting to turn the baby, a procedure that is known as external cephalic version. I believe that it's worth it to try to turn all breeches, because a vaginal breech delivery is a riskier procedure. If your doctor says he or she wants to schedule an external version, this is what will happen:

Usually the procedure will be performed in the hospital. There is a potential for harm to or distress of the baby, so we try to do everything in the safest setting possible. Occasionally, version will result in the need for an emergency C-section, although I've never had that experience as a doctor. Because of the cesarean possibility, we perform versions with an IV already in place, and with the knowledge that there's an operating room available, should we need it. I give the woman a dose of a drug called Terbutaline, a tocolytic which relaxes the uterine muscle and increases my success rate. Then an assistant and I use physical force, pushing on the woman's abdomen and manipulating it, trying to get the baby to do a somersault.

You should know that this is not a pleasant procedure; in fact, it can really hurt. I won't torture a pregnant woman excessively; my feeling is that if the baby's going to turn at all, then it will turn with me and my assistant using our usual strength. If the version fails and the woman ends up needing a cesarean, chances are it will be scheduled for a later date. (See Chapter 10, which focuses exclusively on cesareans.) If you need one, then you need one.

Not all persistent breeches end up being delivered by cesarean. Some can be delivered vaginally, but only if the mother is otherwise in excellent health, if the doctor is *extremely* experienced in this area (ask), and if the baby is small enough or the pelvis large enough for this to be accomplished safely.

As for women carrying twins, the relative positions of the babies to each other often dictate the mode of delivery. If the first baby is head-down, there's an excellent chance for a successful vaginal delivery. If the first baby is breech, however, most doctors would automatically recommend a cesarean. It is also possible that the overdistended uterus just can't generate the necessary force during labor to accomplish a vaginal delivery. For this reason, I strongly encourage these women to consider an epidural in labor because of the increased chances for cesarean section.

CONTRACTIONS AND LABOR

In the final lap of your pregnancy, when you know the big event is going to happen soon, and when most likely you feel extremely ready for it—as in, you can't stand to be pregnant a minute longer, can't stand the constant urinating, the sometimes painful kicking, the trouble breathing—you also may feel, in other ways, extremely unprepared. In spite of the childbirth classes you've been taking, in spite of all the cramming you've done and the conversations you've had with friends who've already gone through it, you feel as though there's something you still don't know, some magical advice you can be given to make it all work out okay. The truth, of course, is that you already know a great deal, and that your body and your doctor and a good labor nurse will help you learn the rest.

One of the most frequently asked questions I hear at the end of a pregnancy is: "How will I know I'm in labor?" For the most part, I can safely say, "You'll know." For first-time mothers, labor tends not to be very subtle. As a rule, actual labor means that the contractions are coming every three to five minutes for the duration of at least an hour. If you or your partner has the presence of mind to time yourself, you'll be able to give your doctor useful information. But if the contractions begin and they're extremely fierce right away—regardless of how close together they are—I feel strongly that a patient shouldn't have to sit at home in the middle of the night in terrible pain.

I have some colleagues who don't like to be called until the three-to-five-minutes-for-an-hour pattern has been established. They know full well that what may feel like labor may just be a dress rehearsal. You may, for example, be contracting every three to five minutes for *half* an hour, then the whole thing may fizzle out into nothing, leaving you feeling bewildered and sheepish. Time will generally sort out the false alarm from the genuine article, but I see no reason for you not to call your doctor if you really are uncomfortable.

When a patient calls me in the middle of the night, I ask her to remind me of her most recent cervical exam, just in case she saw one of my partners at her last visit. If she says, "Oh, Dr. Brodman said the head is low and the cervix is thin," then I know this isn't somebody who should sit at home for too long. With a first baby things generally don't happen quickly, but I've been fooled before. I've had patients whose babies started to crown as the mothers were being wheeled through the labor room door. I remind a patient who lives far from the hospital that if she's waiting in her house and patiently timing contractions before she calls me, she'd better be sure to factor in her travel time. I'd rather have a woman come to the hospital with a false alarm and be sent home, than subject a patient to huffing and puffing in the backseat of a car while the driver speeds along the highway.

If your first contraction is extremely severe, there's no point in staying in bed with a stopwatch, grimly timing yourself through a veil of extreme pain and fear. I tend to send my patients to the hospital on the early side; I'd rather have them on the labor floor for an extra hour or two than sitting at home in the clutches of anxiety. We have anesthesiologists on hand who can offer pain relief, and we have a house staff who can monitor the patients' status.

Some labors kick in with a vengeance, and the sequence of events picks up surprisingly quickly, but others limp along seemingly endlessly. Doctors see labor as broken up into three distinct stages, which are as follows:

1. *The first stage. This includes A) the latent phase, in which there are contractions but not much cervical change and B) the active phase, in which the cervix is changing by at least 1 cm. an hour.*

2. *The second stage, from full dilation of the cervix until delivery, which includes the pushing.*

3. *The third stage, which includes the time between delivery of the baby and delivery of the placenta.*

When your labor begins, you ought to be able to call your doctor in the middle of the night to discuss your situation, without being made to feel that you've called too soon, or unnecessarily.

If any bleeding is suddenly taking place (also called "bloody show"), then you should call right away. Bleeding is indicative of the cervix effacing. If you've got bleeding *and* contractions, chances are you're in labor, and your doctor won't have you hanging around your house for very long.

The passage of the so-called "mucous plug," however, is a different story entirely. The mucous plug is the protective barrier that's been present in the cervix throughout your pregnancy. When it comes out, a woman will notice a thick gob of mucous passing, and in my experience she will become very excited or worried, and call me to tell me about it. But *I* don't get very excited about the loss of a mucous plug; it's not a particularly meaningful event. It just means that the cervix has loosened up enough to drop the plug, and this event can't reliably be used to predict the start of labor. You could lose your plug and then not deliver for two or three weeks. Some women never notice the passage of the plug, and this has no bearing on their progress whatsoever. Women who deliver by cesarean section may never pass a mucous plug, and this too is meaningless. Basically, all that the loosening of the mucous plug tells us is that conditions in the cervix have started to change. This is good to know, but it is *not* information that I need to have in the middle of the night. Bloody show or real labor pains, however, *are* worth waking a doctor.

"But what do labor pains *feel* like?" a patient in her ninth month asked me plaintively the other day. I never did get to experience full labor myself; much to my shock and concern, my membranes ruptured at 32 1/2 weeks and the twins were delivered by C-section. I'd always anticipated going the full nine yards, and was quite disappointed when I didn't, but I think I still have a pretty accurate (if incomplete) understanding of the experience of labor pains from my patients' descriptions.

"Bad menstrual cramps," was the way one woman

described the start of her contractions. "The kind of cramps you used to get in junior high school, and you had to stay home in bed with a heating pad all day." There's a real variation to the way contractions will begin; they might be mild at first and then build, or they might be strong to start with, and grow even stronger. They may start across the belly, or you may experience what is known as "back labor." There is really no way to predict where in your body and exactly how intensely you will experience labor.

I've heard women discuss the particular agony of back labor, but labor is always a very subjective experience, and what is agony for one patient is well tolerated by another. During labor, the entire uterus is squeezing during contractions, and the pain is felt both in back and in front. Some women experience it more in back, and this is loosely classified as back labor. There's a vague but not substantiated theory that the babies of women who have so-called back labor tend to be in the occiput posterior position (which means the baby is sunny-side up, looking at the ceiling instead of the floor). It's hard to know for sure, because by the time most babies have made it all the way down the birth canal, the forces of the contractions will have corkscrewed them into the face-down, easier position for being born.

RUPTURED MEMBRANES

Of course, labor may not be heralded by contractions at all, but may instead be preceded by the rupturing of your membranes (amniotic sac). Ten percent of pregnant women have membranes that rupture before labor. I used to think that when and if a woman's membranes ruptured (a.k.a. "her water broke") she had a good chance of knowing it had happened. Or, at any rate, I felt secure that when and if my water broke, I would know it, having witnessed this wet event so many times in my professional life.

I was wrong. My membranes had been ruptured for 24 hours before I realized it. When it happens, it's a totally painless event. The amniotic sac has literally burst, and what you feel can range from a slow trickle of fluid from your vagina that may lead you to believe it's just another embarrassing moment of incontinence, to a forceful gush reminiscent of Niagara Falls. In my case, my bladder had been behaving pretty well throughout the pregnancy, and I wasn't plagued by the need to go to the bathroom constantly, like so many women.

At week 30+ I was placed on bed rest. One night I felt funny, and initially I thought that my bladder was doing what everyone else always describes. I blithely went through a full day of leakage—going about my business, not paying too much attention to it—until finally the leakage became bloody, and only then did it dawn on me that this was amniotic fluid. It was about 10:30 at night and it all clicked in my mind. I screamed, "Jeff! This has been going on for 24 hours!" We took a cab, even though I live only two blocks from the hospital, because I didn't want to walk in this condition.

If *I* had trouble knowing that my membranes had ruptured, it's not unreasonable to think that you might have trouble knowing, too. If the wetness you feel between your legs feels different from the incontinence you may have been experiencing of late (more copious, or perhaps tinged with blood), then you should contact your doctor right away. He or she may have you brought in to be examined, find that your water has indeed broken, and then, in the absence of contractions, send you home, telling you to return to the hospital in several hours.

If the fluid is stained greenish-brown, this means that there is the presence of something called meconium, which is a bowel movement passed by the baby *in utero*. Meconium staining is serious; it lets us know that the baby has become stressed enough to move its bowels, which babies don't usually do prior to birth. Their intestines generally are not active, but if a baby is being compromised or placed under stress, the anal sphincter relaxes and releases a bowel movement. This signals that there has been some alteration in fetal health. If a woman's membranes rupture and there is meconium present, her doctor will hook her up to a fetal monitor and watch the tracings very closely; in many cases the tracings are normal, but we know that the baby has been stressed at least once before—when the bowel movement was passed—and needs to be observed.

Some women underestimate the volume of amniotic fluid that can leak out during a simple car ride to a doctor's office or hospital. One patient of mine brought about three Kleenex with her in her purse during her taxi ride, and found that these were grossly insufficient and that she had completely drenched the backseat of the cab. (She tipped well.) It might make sense to bring a thick towel with you, and place it between your legs or underneath you. *Never* try to wear a tampon at this time; it can cause infection. A sanitary napkin may prove useless as the fluid continues to spill.

After a woman's membranes have ruptured at term, I know that, one way or another, I will aim to deliver her baby within the next 24 hours, in order to reduce the risk of infection. In a preterm situation, such as the one I found myself in, membranes may rupture but a doctor might decide not to deliver right away, administering prophylactic antibiotics instead to prevent infection and buy more time for the baby to develop.

A pregnant woman may not be able to predict exactly when her baby is going to be born—and each day of waiting may feel like a week—but the flurry of obstetrical visits and excitement and the onset of cervical changes are all indications of the startling proximity of the day of delivery.

Chapter Nine

Showtime

- Induction
- Fetal Monitoring
- Early Labor
- Epidurals
- Pushing
- Forceps
- Episiotomy
- Apgar Scores
- The Placenta

Regardless of whether your contractions have begun or your membranes have ruptured, if your doctor has told you to come to the hospital you will be administered to in the protocol of that particular institution. All hospitals are different, of course. Here's the way things work on most labor floors:

After a patient has been instructed by her doctor to go to the hospital, she'll be greeted at the front desk and shown to a bed in either a triage room or a labor and delivery room; it all depends on how certain her labor really is. (I'd like to add here that a patient should *never* just decide for herself that she's in labor and go off to the hospital without first getting in touch with her doctor. I don't like being surprised by a phone call from a nurse saying, "Um, Dr. Brasner, your patient's here.")

At this point, the patient's intake of food and liquid will be seriously restricted; she probably won't be allowed to ingest anything other than ice chips. This isn't a torture exercise; the main priority is safety, and with the possibility of emergency procedures, an empty stomach is always safer.

If there's any question about whether a patient has really begun laboring or not, she might be checked into triage first. We prefer to keep the labor and delivery beds—which are often in great demand—available. In a triage room, she'll be examined by a member of the house staff or, in some hospitals, a nurse. These exams can sometimes be extremely painful—be forewarned—especially if a woman's cervix is still "unfavorable," that is to say, not soft enough. The exams hurt less as the cervix becomes pliable and easier to examine. The triage staff will get in touch with the doctor after a patient has been examined; this conversation between a resident and a woman's obstetrician will include the resident's observations about the patient's effacement and dilation, as well as the baby's station. If the cervix has registered absolutely no change, then the patient may be sent home.

Being sent home can be greatly disappointing—not to mention irritating—especially if a patient lives far away. I've had women practically bribe hospital staff to be allowed to stay, but the truth is that a labor floor is an active, sometimes overburdened place, and we often can't handle

patients who won't be in need of our services in the immediate future. Still, if a woman is in real pain, I will always
admit her. How can I turn away someone who's crying? I
might offer her a narcotic so she can sleep for a few hours,
during which time her cervix may begin to change. But not
all doctors (or hospitals, for that matter) would agree with
this philosophy. All women know stories of friends who
experienced false alarms; if this happens to you, and you
are "turned away at the inn," as it were, then remind yourself that you will be back soon enough, and that next time it
will most likely be for real.

But if a woman's cervix *has* begun to show some change,
and it's clear that she's truly begun her labor, she will certainly be moved to a labor and delivery room (in some hospitals, these are two separate rooms), which will be hers
until her baby is born. (If for some reason she needs a
cesarean, she will be moved to an operating room, also
called a "section room.") A patient of mine described how,
when she was shown into the labor and delivery room, a
nurse flicked on the lights and said to her, "This is where
it's all going to happen." It seemed astonishing to my
patient that this ordinary little room, with its wallpaper and
reading lamp and television tuned to "The Tonight Show,"
was going to turn into the dramatic place where her baby
would be born.

INDUCTION

If a woman's membranes rupture and her cervix
remains unready for labor for a period of time that's
stretching on too long (to my mind, roughly 24 hours), or if
her contractions seem to be getting her nowhere but into

deeper pain, then there are drugs we can give to jump-start an effective labor. This is called "induction." There are several other reasons for a woman's labor to be induced, including:

- She is past her due date—by at least one to two weeks. (Although in our practice we don't like to let patients go more than 7 to 10 days past their due date.)

- She has a hypertensive disorder or preeclampsia.

- She has diabetes.

- There's the possibility of growth retardation and the uterus is no longer the healthiest environment.

- We have subtle indications that the baby is large. (This is the indication for which there is the least concrete medical justification for inducing labor.)

As for this last reason, I ought to add that with a first baby we never know for sure what's too big for a particular woman's anatomy. If the baby is already too large to pass through the pelvis, then no amount of medication is going to change that. If we arrange to get the baby out a week early, then perhaps we'll improve the mother's chances of delivering vaginally. These decisions are difficult to reach scientifically; basically, a doctor has to be able to trust his or her own instinct.

Many patients actually request to have their labor induced; they often are exhausted, frustrated, anxious, or like knowing when the day of delivery is going to come, and are happy to forgo the surprise onset of labor pains (especially in the middle of the night) and the worries about whether they will reach the hospital on time. Because of the availability of effective induction agents and our experience with their use, we are able to accommodate their wishes. We counsel them about the pros and cons of elective induction, and are willing to proceed after 39 weeks have been completed and the cervix is favorable.

If you were a true medical purist, you might look through my files and conclude that only about 10 percent of our patients absolutely, positively, needed to be induced. The other 15 percent might be said to fall into a gray area; they might have been fine, had we let nature run its course.

Studies do link elective inductions with an increased risk of cesarean sections, but based on my own experience, I don't feel that I'm dramatically altering a woman's outcome when I schedule an induction. My partners and I rely heavily on induction and have a low (15 percent) C-section rate. If induction unconditionally increased the rate of cesareans, I would have a much higher C-section rate. (Again, for more on C-sections, see Chapter Ten.)

Most inductions are performed using the intravenous administration of a drug called oxytocin, which, as I've mentioned, is known by its brand name, Pitocin. ("Pit," in hospital shorthand.) For some reason, women have come to fear this drug. Perhaps Pitocin gots its bad name during the 1970s, when "natural" childbirth (that is, childbirth without the aid of any anesthetic) was de rigueur. It's true that Pitocin will give a woman stronger, more rhythmic contractions that may be more difficult to tolerate without any pain relief. But almost none of my patients—whether on Pitocin or not—opt to go through labor cold-turkey.

We usually don't administer Pitocin on its own if the cervix is uneffaced; instead, if a woman is having a planned induction (meaning we've scheduled the date ahead of time because of one of the reasons mentioned earlier) and her cervix isn't ready, we admit her the night before we give her Pitocin, administering a synthetic form of the chemical prostaglandin into the cervix. This is what a planned induction usually involves:

In the event that the woman's cervix isn't "ripe," the woman enters the hospital the night before the scheduled delivery. She is checked by a member of the house staff, attached to a fetal monitor, and, after a reactive tracing has been obtained, is given a dose of prostaglandin into her vagina. This is a painless procedure, during which a syringeful of gel or a prostaglandin tablet is inserted deep into the vagina. During the night, the house staff will check to see if she's made progress—that is, to see if her cervix has "ripened" at all.

By "ripening," I mean getting softer, more pliant. Think of an unripe cervix as a brick wall. If we were to give a woman Pitocin while her cervix was totally unripe, it would take many, many hours to hack away at those bricks. Now we have the advantage of delivering medication directly into the cervix. As the cervix responds to the stimulus of the prostaglandin, we know that we won't be giving a woman contractions against a brick wall, but against a much softer surface. (There can, in rare cases, be sensitivity and adverse reactions to prostaglandin; occasionally, a woman will have what's known as a "tetanic reaction," in which her uterus contracts and the baby's heartbeat drops considerably. This can be treated quickly by administering Terbutaline, which relaxes the uterus and brings the baby's heartbeat back up to baseline.)

In the morning, if a woman's cervix has responded well, her doctor will administer the Pitocin. (If her cervix was ripe to begin with, this is the point at which her induction begins.) A decision may be made to rupture membranes at this time, because it accelerates the labor process. (For more on membrane rupture, see page 181.) She's attached to an I.V., if she hasn't been already, and as the Pitocin drip slowly enters her bloodstream, she will start to feel contractions. Some women like to have an epidural anesthetic given to them at the same time so that they don't feel the pain of the contractions; different hospitals have their own protocols with regard to how soon a woman can receive an epidural. In some hospitals, an epidural is given only when a woman's cervix is four centimeters dilated or fully effaced. Similarly, some hospitals have a strict cutoff for how late into labor a woman can receive an epidural. If you find out in advance that you're going to be induced, and you think you might like to have pain relief early on, you should talk to your doctor about epidurals before you are admitted to the hospital.

Don't be afraid of Pitocin, but do be prepared for the fact that the contractions that occur may be very intense. I believe that Pitocin is an extremely useful and important drug, in that, in its own tough way, it can not only jump-start but also abbreviate the sometimes seemingly endless process known as labor.

FETAL MONITORING

Once in the room, regardless of whether she's been induced or has gone into labor on her own, a woman's vital signs will be taken, and she will give one final urine sample so that it can be dipped for protein. Then she will likely be attached to a fetal monitor.

If a woman has already had non-stress tests in her doctor's office, she knows what fetal monitoring entails, but if she hasn't, here's a brief recap for you: A nurse will hand her a "belt," which is made of very stretchy tube-top material. The patient will slip it over her head and get into bed. Then the nurse will apply gel to the patient's belly and attach two small, disk-shaped monitors. One of these is the uterine activity monitor, and the other is the fetal heart monitor. The stretchy belt is pulled down over the monitors, keeping them securely in place. The fetal monitor itself—the small Doppler machine to which she'll be attached—gives a beat-by-beat printout of the baby's heartbeat, as well as a record of uterine activity.

At our hospital, the patient will stay attached to the fetal monitor for the duration of the labor and delivery. Some hospitals do only intermittent monitoring, but I'm much more comfortable having a continuous look at how often the contractions are coming, and what the baby's heartrate response looks like on a printout. If the baby's heartbeat drops, we'll know it by reading the numbers on the monitor. Even if a doctor or nurse isn't in the room, the readout on the monitor is usually transmitted on a TV screen at the nurses' station, so someone will see it.

I've had patients who initially complain about the continuous monitor, telling me that they read in a book that it was better to get up and walk around during labor. A midwife or less conservative doctor may be in favor of intermittent fetal monitoring. In the long run, however, I think my patients ultimately are grateful for the chance to stay in bed and take it easy. The hard work of pushing still lies ahead. I want a fetal monitor on all of my patients; you should want one on you, too.

Another form of monitoring that might be employed later on in delivery is called the "fetal scalp monitor," or an "internal" monitor, which isn't routine but is sometimes necessary. This is a thin wire that's inserted vaginally (and painlessly) and attached to the baby's scalp, in the event that the fetal monitor shows an abnormal tracing and we need further clarification of how the baby is tolerating labor. The fetal scalp monitor gives us more information by assessing what is known as "beat to beat" variability, and helps rule out fetal distress.

An even more aggressive form of fetal assessment is a scalp pH sample. We might use this tool in labor if the baby displays an ominously low heartrate, or if there's any meconium in the amniotic fluid, either of which indicate that the baby is under a certain degree of stress. The scalp pH sample helps us assess exactly how stressed the baby is. We can perform this test only if the mother's membranes have ruptured (either on their own or through the doctor's doing), her cervix is dilated, and the baby's head is accessible enough for us to reach in and take a scalp sample. A conelike structure is put into the woman's vagina, which assists in visualizing the fetal head. An instrument that has a tiny razor on the end of it is used to nick the baby's scalp. One drop of blood is automatically dripped into a glass tube. Then we take the blood and put it in a machine elsewhere on the labor floor, which gives us a readout of the pH of the baby's blood. The pH measures the acid-base balance within the blood; the normal range is 7.25–7.35. If a baby's pH is lower than that, we know that this is a baby who can no longer compensate for a decreased oxygen supply and whose well-being is becoming compromised. When the pH drops, acid accumulates in the blood, and we

need to consider delivery in the next few minutes if there is
no improvement.

EARLY LABOR

But for now, at the beginning of labor, we are far away
from making those kinds of decisions. While the patient is
being settled in her room, the member of the house staff
who examined her will discuss with the doctor when he or or
she needs to arrive on the scene. A woman's doctor may be
required to be present for the administration of Pitocin, as
well as for epidural anesthetics. But a doctor doesn't need to
be present during the phase of labor that is considered prodromal, or latent. This means early labor, in which the
patient is contracting but the cervix isn't changing much.

We know from experience that the latent phase can last a
long, long time in women who have not been given any
augmenting drugs: up to 20 hours for a first baby is normal, and up to 12 hours is normal for subsequent babies. In
some hospitals, she will be sent home during this latent
phase; other places will send her home with a low-dose
sedative. I like to keep my patients in the hospital if they're
uncomfortable, and help them with pain relief. I require a
woman to be hooked up to a fetal monitor if she's receiving
any sort of pain medication. Obviously, if she's walking
around fairly comfortably, then she doesn't yet need either
pain relief or fetal monitoring. If a woman is, however, in
pain and agitated, I'll give her the option of being sedated
with a mild narcotic, usually meperidine (Demerol). I'm
wary of the usage of narcotics during labor, as are most of
my patients; these drugs do cross the placenta and can
sedate the baby as well as the mother. But in the prodromal

phase I find that a woman can be aided by taking a very
light dose of Demerol, which will not compromise her
baby. A little Demerol allows her to sleep through these
early contractions, and save her energy for later. Without it,
she might lie awake in pain, becoming needlessly keyed up
and increasingly uncomfortable. Also, narcotics actually
have a therapeutic effect, and can help the cervix melt away
faster. I don't use Demerol all that often, but if I think it's
going to be a long prodromal phase and a woman accepts it,
it can be very useful. Because the prodromal phase tends to
go on for a matter of hours, by the time the woman reaches
what we call "active" labor (the later stages in which there is
progressive cervical change) the effects of the Demerol will
certainly have worn off on both mother and baby.

In rare situations, a woman is given some Demerol and
sleeps for a little while, only to awaken and find herself in
active labor much sooner than we'd calculated. The baby, in
these cases, might be born sluggish from Demerol; if this
happens, we immediately give the baby a shot of Narcan, a
drug that reverses the effects of narcotics. But it's rare for
this to happen. In all my deliveries, I think I've had to give a
shot of Narcan only twice.

At some point, a patient may have an IV placed in her
arm. This hurts for a few seconds as a nurse or doctor finds
the vein, but it allows us to speedily give her any medications or fluids she may need over the course of the delivery.
I don't want to fumble while searching for a vein in an
emergency situation later, frantically trying to insert a needle. I'd rather have it taken care of ahead of time.

My patients often have some misconceptions about giving
birth. They have images of being forced to take enemas, or
having their pubic hair shaved. Neither of these practices is

widely used anymore. (If either one is still used at your hospital, you might ask if you can skip it.) Sometimes, women actually *ask* me for an enema, because they've heard stories of patients having bowel movements in labor, and the idea is so mortifying to them that they want their intestines emptied beforehand. I tell them that I've seen women excreting all kinds of things in labor: bowel movements, vomit, blood, and babies, and that if nothing embarrasses me, *they* shouldn't be embarrassed, either. Women can also have an erroneous view of what the atmosphere in a labor room will be like; they sometimes imagine that the entire time spent there will be dramatic and noisy and nerve-racking, like a delivery in a Hollywood movie. But in actuality, most deliveries are fairly calm and quite boring for long stretches of time. There's a lot of waiting around, a lot of hanging out during the prodromal phase until something concrete starts to happen and the active phase begins.

Once it's clear that a patient is making cervical progress—and this includes induced patients—we like to rupture the membranes, if this hasn't already taken place on its own. Breaking the water (also called amniotomy) accelerates labor. It is a painless procedure, although the vaginal exam that accompanies it will probably be painful, so be prepared. An amniotomy involves the usage of an instrument called an amnio hook, which is basically a long stick with a little curve at the end that's as sharp as a pin. We insert the hook vaginally until it pricks the membranes, rupturing them as though breaking a balloon. Once we've done this, what follows may happen quickly, or else it may unravel in a long, drawn-out manner, causing the doctor to suggest starting the patient on Pitocin to help shorten the labor phase.

As I mentioned earlier in this chapter, Pitocin gives a

woman more intense and rhythmically predictable contractions, which can become unmanageably painful. Whether
she's been given Pitocin or not, I want my patients to have
all the facts about the pain management that is available
during delivery, especially about one method in particular:
the epidural.

EPIDURALS

Whenever I've glanced at a pregnancy advice book that one
of my patients has brought into the office, I've been surprised
at the way epidurals tend to be treated. They're often mentioned almost casually in a group of possibilities, as though
they're just another decent option that a woman might—but
only might—end up wanting during delivery.

I happen to believe the epidural is God's gift to pregnant
women. Every woman should at least be given the option to
have one.

The name "epidural" refers to the place where the anesthetic medication actually goes—in this case into the "epidural
space" in the spine. In the past year, only two of my patients
have chosen to labor without an epidural. The epidural is to
labor what the Pill originally was to sex: It's revolutionized the
experience entirely. I firmly believe that no woman should
have to labor without one if she doesn't want to. After all, what
other operation or invasive medical procedure would a patient
be expected to undergo without anesthesia? Doctors don't say
to patients, when they're about to perform an appendectomy,
"Now, you have the option of some anesthesia, if you'd prefer.
Or you could try it without anesthesia." They simply *give* the
patient the anesthetic, knowing that all patients will "want" it.

The grandmothers and great-aunts of my patients argue

that they themselves labored differently, and they don't understand why laboring women today want these drugs. I think I can address their puzzlement: Because an epidural can help a woman actually enjoy labor, participate in the birth of her child in a positive and painless way. And it's much easier for the husband or birth partner to be part of the experience if the mother isn't hysterical.

Still, there are some women who honestly want to labor "without anything." This is a personal decision and I do respect it, but I always like to make sure that a patient isn't choosing to have a totally drug-free delivery out of some need to prove to herself or someone else that she can, or else out of some outdated fear that I might easily be able to allay by giving her further information.

If the only alternative to pain in delivery were a general anesthetic, as it was in the old days, I would probably encourage women to stay awake and try to cope with the pain. General anesthesia isn't a good idea in delivery, and should only be used in emergencies. But today we are fortunate to have another option. Epidurals are terrific in that they let you remain fully awake and have your wits about you while you push out your baby. As I said, I respect the decision of women who elect to endure childbirth without an epidural, although I can't say I fully understand it. But it's not my place to plumb the psyches or the pain thresholds of my patients.

Some women who initially say they don't want an epidural will choose one ultimately when confronted with real—not theoretical—pain. Certain childbirth classes will encourage women to "determine" their pain thresholds, in order to see whether or not they will be able to tough it out during labor. In my opinion, no woman's pain threshold has ever been high enough to make labor seem like mild cramps. The pain of childbirth is profound, and it can go on and on. But with an epidural, it doesn't have to. If I had had a vaginal delivery, there's no question in my mind that I would have requested an epidural as soon as I felt uncomfortable.

Of course, this is only one opinion, and I don't know your particular circumstances. Be sure to discuss the matter with your doctor prior to being admitted into the hospital. In rare cases, as mentioned earlier, a woman won't be permitted to receive an epidural because she has a coagulation disorder, and the anesthesiologist wouldn't want to stick a needle into her back. Also, a woman who's had extensive back surgery or a history of scoliosis may not be able to receive one.

Occasionally a woman wants an epidural but is told that it's too late. (The only real missed window of opportunity occurs when the patient is too far along in her labor, in which case she's pretty much home free anyway.) There are cases, however, when a patient is fully dilated but it's clear she still has a long pushing phase ahead of her. In these instances, I'm not opposed to administering an epidural to help her get through this tough time. Although you may have been frightened by stories of women missing out on epidurals, rest assured that most first labors aren't quick, and are in fact prolonged events in which there is plenty of time for the administering of an epidural.

Although I'm not doctrinaire about exactly when a patient can receive an epidural, I'm not a big fan of administering one when the cervix is still uneffaced and closed. There is still a great distance to cover in the latent phase, and some studies indicate that an epidural can prolong this phase. I might instead suggest that the patient receive a narcotic at this point, so she can get the pain relief she needs. Intravenous narcotics are good for the latent phase, but less good, as I've indicated, for the active phase. An epidural is far and above better than a narcotic during the active phase of labor, because it will have no negative effects on the baby (and because the patient won't miss the most exciting part!).

The "best" time to ask for an epidural is when you really want one, which, in most cases, means when your contractions have become painful and your cervix is beginning to show some change. You don't have to be writhing in agony, merely very uncomfortable. If your hospital has a full-time anesthesia staff, you'll be able to get an epidural when you want it, but if it doesn't, then you may have to wait awhile, possibly in real discomfort. These are the sort of details that you ought to figure out now, before you check into the hospital.

This is how an epidural is administered: First, the father or birth partner may be asked to leave the room. Sometimes they can get pretty squeamish at the sight of the needle, and we really don't want to have to deal with fainting or panic attacks at this moment. The mother is also hooked up to an I.V., if she hasn't been already. This fluid protects against a possible drop in blood pressure associated with epidurals and allows for the administration of medicines to improve the blood pressure, in the event it does indeed drop.

Next, she will be asked to sit up in bed and lean forward; at our hospital, we have the woman lean across a table that is wheeled up close to the bed. As she leans over, her lower back is swabbed with an antibacterial agent such as Betadine, which will feel cold. Then the skin is anesthetized. The place for the injection—somewhere in the lower part of the spine—

is located, and the doctor will insert the needle. There's often a feeling of slightly unpleasant pressure as the needle goes in—entering the spine until it reaches the layer called the epidural space. Then the doctor threads a very narrow tube through the needle, removes the needle and tapes the tubing to the woman's back so that it stays in place as long as it's needed. It's important for the patient to remain motionless throughout the placement of the epidural and to let the anesthesiologist know when contractions are coming. The anesthesia staff are used to working between contractions in order to have the patient keep perfectly still. (Sometimes women worry: *What if I move?* But the placement is brief, and the vast majority of women do fine.) Sometimes there's a brief sting from the anesthetic. As the drug enters the spine, it bathes the whole area in local anesthetic.

The key to administering an epidural is to bring the level up slowly, in order to minimize the possibility of a blood-pressure drop. Essentially, once you ask for an epidural it takes about 15 minutes for doctors and nurses to prep and drape you and get the catheter into place, then another 15 minutes for the drug to be administered. All in all, therefore, pain relief will arrive approximately half an hour after the procedure begins. As the anesthetic begins to take effect, a woman's torso and legs will grow numb. She will be able to move them, but the sensation will be a bit strange. Anesthetics always feel peculiar; if you've ever had Novocaine at the dentist, then you know the feeling.

The epidural stays in place and can be constantly replenished throughout labor, no matter how long the process lasts. At our hospital, you receive a couple of initial doses called "boluses," and then you're on a low-dose continuous infusion to avoid the breakthrough of pain. I generally don't shut that drip off even for pushing. For the most part, the sensation of pressure on the rectum is still present, and a woman is able (with coaching) to be an effective pusher. An epidural *does* make it harder to push, and pushing often takes longer, but I'd rather have a pain-free labor followed by an hour and a half of pushing, instead of an excruciating labor followed by an hour's worth of pushing. And when the baby is born, if the woman needs an episiotomy, she's already got an anesthetic on board, and won't even feel the incision or stitches.

I am often asked whether there are any real risks associated with an epidural. My patients tell me they've heard horror stories about women becoming permanently paralyzed. I want to stress that neurological complications are quite rare. Performed correctly—all anesthesiologists should be well-versed in the procedure—an epidural is extremely safe.

The advantages of an epidural definitely outweigh the disadvantages, as far as I'm concerned. Those theoretical disadvantages mentioned in medical studies largely concern the links between epidural use and longer labors, increased cesarean sections, and higher costs. I believe it's quite difficult to interpret these studies. There are so many confounding variables; the patients are all different, as is the size of their babies. Some interesting studies indicate that there's been a misinterpretation of the "epidural and increased cesarean risk" link. These studies suggest that women who have a long latent phase, or women who experience intense pain very early on, are giving a signal that their bodies aren't going to labor successfully no matter what. It's as though these women may have a certain predisposition that is going to make it more likely for them to have cesareans.

The only negative I have to say about epidurals is that they can, very occasionally, lead to a crushing headache, which usually kicks in the following day. (This happens to 1 in 100 women.) Because an epidural needle is thicker than a spinal tap needle, if it goes in too far it can leave a woman with spinal fluid leakage and a profound headache, also called a "post-dural puncture headache." Although these headaches are agonizing, they are not life-threatening and can resolve on their own. We treat this problem with conservative measures such as Tylenol, intravenous hydration, and with another epidural placement, into which we inject the patient's own blood. Her blood actually patches the hole, seals it, and there's no longer any fluid leaking. I know 1 in 100 aren't the world's greatest odds, but I still encourage a woman to get an epidural if she's inclined in that direction. A headache can be remedied, and the woman will still have had a much more pleasurable labor.

In most cases, an epidural is a miracle procedure that has transformed the way many women go through one of the most profound experiences of their lives.

PUSHING

Much of labor can seem quite humdrum, especially if a woman has been given an epidural. As I've already said, the latent phase (in which a woman has contractions but her cervix isn't undergoing any progressive change), can take as long as 20 hours in a first-time mother, and the active phase (in which the cervix changes by at least one centimeter an hour) can take up to six hours. You never know when you'll get to the active phase until, suddenly, you're there. In many cases, the real drama, if there's going to be any, takes place during pushing. This is a part of delivery that women either hate or love, usually depending on whether they've had a previous baby. My patients tell me that they've read in other books how "rewarding" pushing can be after all that waiting. I have to warn you that many first-time mothers find pushing a difficult, even horrible, experience. No matter how much they practiced in childbirth class, holding their breaths until they were purple in the face (not an effective method, by the way), it's a whole different ballgame once they're doing it for real.

Women who have had previous babies (known in short-hand as "multips") have a much, much easier time of it than "primips" (first time mothers). The length of time it takes a woman to push her first baby out is generally between one and two hours. For a second baby, it's usually a fraction of this time. It's as though, with second babies, the body finally knows what to do on its own, and the way has been paved (with great difficulty, I might add) by baby number one.

Because pushing can be harrowing for a first-time mother, the involvement and encouragement of the doctor, labor nurse, and birth partner are essential. Almost all of an obstetrician's tasks during a woman's pregnancy are purely medical: checking urine and blood sugar, listening to the heartbeat, etc. But during pushing, an obstetrician (and everyone else in the room) needs to help the patient get into the right psychological frame of mind. Women need positive reinforcement during the task of pushing; they need to know when the pushes they've made are effective, so that they can repeat them. All doctors have different styles, of course, but I tend to push right along with my patients, holding one of the legs and encouraging her as we count together. Sometimes I feel like a cheerleader waving pom-

poms, egging that baby on, and my obvious enthusiasm seems to help the mother rise to the occasion.

My way of thinking about pushing is that a woman should push *only* during contractions. As the contraction starts to come (and a woman will either be able to feel it or, in the absence of sensation due to anesthetic, will learn about it from the tracing on the fetal monitor), she should give her first push while holding her breath and while the doctor or labor nurse counts out loud from one to ten. On "ten," she should release the breath and quickly take another, going through the process again, and then yet again during the same contraction. That means I want to see three good pushes with each contraction. There will be enough time to accomplish all of this; the average contraction at this stage of labor lasts about one minute.

Sometimes, observing the crest of the contraction on the monitor (even if she already feels the pain or pressure rising) can provide additional "focusing" on the moment, allowing the woman to know exactly when she is going to need to take that big breath. It's similar to "jumping in" during a game of jump rope, or leaping onto a wave while body surfing.

As the woman sees her contraction rise, I will say to her, "Okay, take a slow, deep, cleansing breath. Now hold it, and push! 2, 3, 4, 5, 6, 7, 8, 9, 10. . . . Now let it out." On the monitor, by the end of the third such episode of holding her breath, pushing and counting, she will see the hill of the contraction returning to the baseline, and will begin to understand the pattern of contractions, and her own role in pushing during them.

What I try to accomplish during the pushing stage is to help a woman focus her energy *away* from her face.

Misdirecting their energy is a common error that first-time mothers make during pushing; they feel confident that they're doing everything right, and they give it all they've got, but their pushes are fruitless. I can't tell you how many times I've witnessed a patient perched on the bed with her face dark red, her cheeks puffed way out, looking like an illustration of the North Wind in a children's storybook. While it all appears very impressive up above, the force isn't being put to use down below. All that effort is wasted if it's not being focused on the right place.

Always keep in mind that the biggest part of the baby is the head; I tell women that if they can focus on the baby's head, they will direct the force to exactly where it's needed. (I usually locate the baby's head with my fingers to orient them.) The harder and more effective a woman makes each push, the less time overall she'll actually spend pushing.

I've seen women who, between pushes, like to chat with their partners, or schmooze with the nurse and doctor, but I prefer that they keep still and rest, even closing their eyes for the couple of minutes they have before the next contraction begins. If there was ever a time to take it easy, this between-contractions interlude is it. The longer the pushing lasts, the more women innately understand the need to rest, and the room seems to grow infinitely quieter and calmer as they close their eyes and try to completely relax, before having to marshal all their energy for the next round of pushing.

I find that it often helps to tell women to try and mimic the sensation of being constipated. If they focus on the rectum, they will more effectively move the baby's head down the birth canal. Some women benefit from a little rectal pressure; the obstetrician or the nurse can put a couple of fingers in the woman's vagina and press down toward the rectum as a way of helping the patient redirect her energy. Fairly often, this kind of intense pushing will produce not a baby at first, but a bowel movement. This is no big deal and is simply wiped away.

Some women like to have a mirror strategically placed, so that they can see the baby as it finally emerges. Then again, other women find that the mirror image is confusing, that it actually throws their concentration off a little.

This is it: We're almost there. The mood in the delivery room at this point palpably elevates. For the mother, the hard part is just about over, and the reward for all the work of the last nine months—all the watching and waiting and, sometimes, worrying—is quite literally within reach. For the medical staff, including the doctor, the delivery of a baby is, in a sense, a routine occurrence, nothing that any one of us doesn't see several times a week, if not several times a day. During one memorable 24-hour period—a New Year's Eve, as it happened—I delivered *four* babies. And yet . . . and yet these final seconds always carry a charge. Call it adrenaline, call it release, or call it simple awe, but whatever it is, it's always present at this last stage of the delivery. And I do mean always—even during every last one of those four New Year's Eve births.

At the very end, I have a woman stop pushing, so I can control the delivery. I now perform something called a Ritgen maneuver, in which I apply pressure upward from behind the rectum, pushing the baby's head up and over the perineum (the area between the rectum and the vagina). I don't mean to pat myself on the back too much, but I'm pretty skilled at this maneuver, and as a result I've helped many patients avoid an episiotomy, which is an inci-

sion made in the perineum in order to increase the circumference of the vagina. The slower and more controlled the
delivery of the head, the less chance a woman has of tearing
or extending her episiotomy. As the baby's head emerges, I
lift it up behind the chin very, very slowly; I consider this
my "technique," and it really works for me.

Men are typically wowed by the sight of their baby's head
emerging from a woman's body; it often makes them feel
overwhelmed. I like to involve the father as much as possible during the delivery, letting him know everything I'm
doing and making sure he sees the top of the baby's head;
it's good for him to know how close he is to actually being a
father—not to mention the fact that it gives him an appreci-
ation of what the woman has been going through. After the
baby has been delivered, I usually ask him if he wants to cut
the umbilical cord. I've had one or two men faint when their
babies were born, but for the most part everyone in the room
performs well, rising fully to the occasion—father, mother,
and baby.

FORCEPS

Sometimes pushing isn't as productive as I might have
hoped, and a woman really knocks herself out over the
course of an hour or two yet finds herself ultimately unable
to dislodge the baby. It's as though there's an imaginary
hump inside—a ledge, a stumbling block, a log in the
road—that the baby just can't overcome. Our goal is to
deliver a healthy baby, and sometimes women are simply
unable to push a baby out on their own, or the heartrate
tracing indicates a situation in which a faster delivery may
help avoid fetal distress. At this point, I might reassess the

situation—taking into account how exhausted the mother is, and how long she's been laboring—and offer her some additional help in the form of forceps.

Whenever the word "forceps" is mentioned toward the end of labor, many patients automatically recoil and say "Oh, no, not those!" They've heard so many bad stories about forceps' usage, stories that have linked them to brain damage or disfiguring, permanent marks on the baby's forehead. While it's true that forceps can inflict harm if used incorrectly or carelessly, a doctor who is skilled in their use can give a woman the assistance in delivery that she may well need. It's important to remember that we doctors want to deliver healthy babies too; we'll do everything within reason to avoid delivering babies with birth trauma or cerebral palsy. I sometimes find myself telling a patient that I haven't taken care of her for these entire nine months to throw it all out the window now.

Forceps are comprised of two separate halves, which look like a pair of broken salad tongs with long, curved blades. We apply each blade separately and then lock them together once they are in place. The forceps are applied to the maxillary prominences on the baby (roughly under eye level, between cheekbone and jawbone). A doctor helps flex and apply traction to the fetal head to accomplish delivery. A telltale "forceps mark" that is left behind will usually disappear within 24 hours.

Forceps have fallen out of favor in recent years, largely because doctors are less willing to put themselves in risky situations with a malpractice potential. But if your doctor is comfortable and confident with forceps (and you might want to address this issue directly prior to delivery), and a situation arises that warrants the need, I don't think you should be frightened. If I had delivered my twins vaginally and had some difficulty at the end, it would have been fine with me had my doctor offered forceps.

Recently I had the satisfaction of delivering twins, both via forceps. The mother had pushed for two hours, but still hadn't delivered. The nurses had the O.R. set up for a cesarean section in the event that the forceps didn't help, but the whole procedure turned out to be a piece of cake, the twins were born with ease, and everyone was happy to avoid surgery.

EPISIOTOMY

As mentioned earlier, an episiotomy is an incision designed to increase the circumference of the vaginal opening. As you may vaguely remember from ninth-grade math class, the circumference of a circle is $2\pi r$ ("r" meaning "radius"). An episiotomy increases the "r." The decision to perform an episiotomy is essentially made at the last minute. I need to see how much the woman's skin stretches over the baby's crowning vertex. The episiotomy rate is definitely lower in multips, who tend to have more elasticity in the region, but this isn't to say that I routinely cut episiotomies in all first-time mothers, and neither should your doctor. In fact, I work very hard to avoid episiotomies, and so do most of the obstetricians I know. However, most doctors would rather repair a small, clean surgical cut than a jagged perineal tear, which is the alternative if the skin is stretched too far.

There are two kinds of episiotomies. If you picture the face of a clock, a "median" incision enters at the 6 o'clock position. A "mediolateral" incision enters at 4 o'clock or 8 o'clock. The decision to make one type of incision instead of the other is usually based on the doctor's preference. After the baby is delivered, the incision is sewn up with absorbable stitches. As I've already mentioned, I find that a very slow and controlled delivery of the baby's head increases the odds that the woman won't need an episiotomy. But if she does, chances are that the epidural will already be in place, and the procedure itself won't hurt much. Extensions of an episiotomy can involve the rectum, which needs special care during repair to maintain the function of the anal sphincter.

The recovery from an episiotomy may be the hard part. The stitches tend to itch and generally feel uncomfortable as the days pass, but eventually the thread dissolves on its own. If you are in real pain, though (and you might not be; some women find an episiotomy recovery no big deal), it can be treated with anesthetic creams, ice packs, witch-hazel pads, and pain relievers, as well as something called a peri-care bottle—a squeeze bottle you fill with warm soapy water to cleanse the area. It's much less abrasive than toilet paper, and can be extremely soothing. If the nurses don't give you one, you might want to request it.

Remember that even without an episiotomy, most women experience soreness as a result of the passage of a seven- or eight-pound baby. An episiotomy increases that discomfort, certainly, but sometimes it can't be avoided. With or without an episiotomy, childbirth is traumatic, but the vagina heals remarkably quickly. Intercourse itself often traumatizes the vagina, but as time passes it heals. (If it were up to me, I would never have put the organs where they are. In my opinion, the rectum and the vagina have no business being so close together.) The only consolation I can offer is that an episiotomy can really hurt, but it will heal more quickly than almost any other bodily incision you're likely to have done.

APGAR SCORES

The obstetrician and labor nurse usually take care of a baby in the first moments after an uneventful birth. After the head has been delivered but not the body, we suction out the baby's nasal passages and mouth with a simple aspiration bulb, in order to clear secretions. If the amniotic fluid is meconium-stained, we use a longer, narrower tube to suction any meconium that may be at or below the vocal cords. It's really important to do this before the baby takes a deep breath and potentially aspirates meconium into his or her lungs. After the aspiration has been completed and the umbilical cord has been cut, the baby finally can be handed over to the mother.

As you can well imagine, this is truly one of the more overwhelming moments in life. It's often a time for tears; I've even been known to wipe away a few of my own, usually in response to the patient's own display of emotion. Some women put their newborns on the breast right away for a couple of moments of sucking practice; this kind of close-ness is good for both mother and baby, especially because it may be a while before the baby is returned to the mother.

The labor nurse now transforms into a baby nurse, cleaning the newborn and putting antibiotic ointment into its eyes to protect against infection. If you haven't spent any time around babies when they've just come into the world, be prepared for the fact that they often look some-what odd. They rarely present the appealing rosiness of babies in movies; those onscreen "newborns" are usually weeks old. (Who in their right mind would let a day-old or even a week-old baby go to work on a movie set?) Here are a few of the details that you might observe in your new baby as you give him or her the tearful once-over:

• **Unusual color.** There's a wide range of appearance at birth, regardless of race or the skin tone of the baby's parents. Babies range from surprisingly pale to surprisingly purple. All of this is completely normal, and coloration changes as the baby gets older.

• **Molding of the head.** A newborn baby often has a strangely-shaped head, which represents the accommodation of that head to the maternal bony pelvis. A related manifestation is something known as caput, which is the swelling of the soft tissue of the head. Molding and caput together can conspire to give the baby that "coneheaded" look that many parents are dismayed to observe. Don't worry; it all recedes soon enough—the caput within days, the molding within a couple of weeks. But, believe me, it can look quite extreme in the beginning.

• **Lanugo.** This is a fine layer of body hair (sometimes dark) that can lend the baby a slightly furry, marsupial look. It usually disappears in the first days or weeks.

• **Vernix.** How brilliant your baby is to know that he or she needs a moisturizer. The presence of the cheesy white substance known as vernix prevents skin damage and wrinkling to a baby who's been floating in a continuous bath for many months.

If we know in advance that a baby is likely to have some physical problems that need attention, then we will arrange to have a pediatrician standing by in the room at the time of birth. And if a baby is born and we suddenly find that there is an unexpected complication, we can have a pediatrician arrive immediately. (At our hospital there are intercoms that connect us directly with Pediatrics, which is one floor above us.) Basically, my job is to be present for the mother, and Pediatrics is there for the baby. In certain situations a baby might be sent to the special care nursery to be observed: if a baby is very small, for example, or if a woman has been given magnesium sulfate or a narcotic just before delivery (in order to ensure the baby doesn't have a reaction to the drug). New mothers often become very upset if the baby is sent to the special care nursery, but I reassure them it's no cause for alarm. The pediatricians tend to be quite conservative in their approach, and in most cases are just playing it safe.

Most babies, however, don't need a pediatrician around within those first minutes after birth. Some do need to be stimulated a little, in order to improve their color or to get them to emit a first, lusty cry. As the labor nurse assesses a baby (first at one minute after birth, then again at five minutes), she will "grade" him or her in several categories, assigning a 0, 1, or 2 in each of the following categories: appearance (color), pulse, reflexes, muscle tone, and respiration. A total score of 7 or better is desirable. Most healthy babies get an 8 or a 9. On the labor floor where I work, newborns usually lose one point for color, and pretty much need to be walking and talking in order to score a 10.

THE PLACENTA

The placenta is delivered, on the average, within five minutes after the baby, although the procedure can take up to thirty minutes. (It's often called, appropriately, the "after-birth.") Sometimes doctors become impatient if they have to wait around too long for this anticlimactic moment. Once the baby has been delivered, the real ordeal is over, and the arrival of the placenta is usually a non-event. There's a gush of blood as the placenta separates from the mother, then a sensation of pressure. It resembles a big piece of liver and has a membranous sac attached. By this point, it may have turned inside-out, which often happens as it is delivered, but I'm happy to re-create it for a patient, to show her exactly how perfectly it nourished her baby all these months.

Most placentas deliver intact, although doctors do need to examine them to see if there are any tears in the membrane, which might indicate that a piece has been left in the uterus. It's important that no placental material remains inside the woman, because such a situation can cause bleeding and infection. Also, a uterus that's not completely empty can't contract well and return to its prepregnancy size.

Following a delivery, a baby will be brought up to the nursery for evaluation by a pediatrician. During this time, a woman will either recover in the labor and delivery room, or be brought to the recovery room for a couple of hours, before being wheeled, still on a bed, to a room on the post-partum floor.

I'm often asked if I am excited when I deliver babies, or whether it's become routine and humdrum by now. The answer is that I am definitely excited, and often moved. Recently I delivered the baby of a couple who had previously experienced a 33-week loss *in utero*—one of those *extremely* rare and sad occurrences—and right up until the moment the new baby came out, the husband and wife were nervous. When I handed this woman the baby, I said to her, "Now you can wash all your fears away."

I think this is true, to some extent, of every pregnant woman. We all worry that something will go wrong, and those worries never entirely disappear until that moment when the baby draws its first breath, and the new mother lets out her own long and well-earned breath of relief.

Chapter Ten

And Now, a Few Words about Cesareans

- Common Reasons for Surgery
- The Procedure
- Recovery

The chapter on cesareans is usually the section in a pregnancy book that most women will quickly glance at but don't want to concentrate on. There's almost a superstitious quality at work here, as though a woman thinks that if she learns too much about cesareans, she may in fact end up needing one. Often, when a labor doesn't go as planned and I have to perform a cesarean, my patient seems to know almost nothing about the procedure, because, like most women, she's kept herself in the dark.

I am here to say, as both a doctor and someone who has undergone the surgery herself: Learn a little bit about the procedure, just in case. I'm not saying you need to bone up on all the specifics, but I do think it helps to know a little about what it entails, in the event that your doctor decides that you need one. A bit of knowledge will help prepare you for what you might experience, and will help make you less frightened.

Contrary to what many patients think, a cesarean isn't a terrible experience. It's a lot easier to recover from a vaginal delivery, of course, but the way cesareans are performed today allows for a much quicker recovery than from cesareans of the not-so-distant past. Abdominal surgery is never pleasant, and I do everything possible to prevent women from having to undergo it. But cesareans are a fact of life. Nationally, 22% of all births are by cesarean. The number is significant enough for me to want my patients to understand a little bit about the procedure in advance. So it might do you some good to take a moment to educate yourself. Then you can hurriedly turn the page.

COMMON REASONS FOR SURGERY

There are several situations in which a doctor may have no choice but to perform a cesarean, either as a scheduled event or else after an unforeseen complication has suddenly precipitated it. Reasons for the increased likelihood of a cesarean can include the following:

• **Breech** position. As mentioned earlier, so-called "breech babies" make for risky vaginal deliveries. There is a higher complication rate for breeches born vaginally, partly due to the fact that premature babies are more likely to be breech. The baby's head—the largest part of the body—is delivered last. Because vaginal breech births have more potential to cause fetal harm, they require an obstetrician who is very comfortable performing such a delivery, and has had a lot of experience with breeches before.

In my practice, we have strict criteria for considering a breech to be delivered vaginally, and these include:

1. *That the baby isn't a first baby, and the mother has delivered vaginally before.* (That way, we know that at least *some* baby fit through.)

2. *That the baby is a frank breech* (buttocks first, not feet first).

3. *That the fetal weight is average, and the baby is neither too small nor too big.*

If a baby doesn't meet these criteria, then a cesarean will probably be scheduled. Try to look at it this way: There's something to be said for a planned delivery, even a surgical one. You know exactly when it's coming and what it will entail. If you need to psych yourself up for it—or calm yourself down—you'll be able to do so in plenty of time. You can also make plans more easily, knowing that you're going to be in the hospital longer than the vaginal delivery patient (who, thanks to recent legislation designed to reduce so-called "drive-through" deliveries, is now entitled to 48 hours in the hospital after the baby is born), and that you will need time at home to recover afterward.

• **Twins and triplets.** Despite what you may have heard, it's *not* automatic that twins will be delivered by C-section. The relative position of the babies tends to dictate the course of action. If twin A isn't head down, then a C-section is safer, regardless of the position of twin B. If both babies are head-down and a good size, we can often perform a safe vaginal delivery. Triplets, however, are delivered by cesarean section

99 percent of the time. They are always small babies, and a cesarean gives us greater control over the delivery.

• **Placenta previa.** With this medical condition, as I mentioned on page 87, the placenta covers the cervix, which is the baby's exit from the womb. This makes it difficult to deliver the baby without disrupting the blood supply—a situation that would endanger both mother and baby—so a cesarean is always the right course of action.

• **Protracted labor.** All labors feel frustratingly long and difficult to the women who are experiencing them, but doctors know the difference between a regular, productive labor and one that goes on too long without making progress. A baby that for some reason can't make it through the birth canal (reasons may include macrosomia, small maternal pelvis, an infection in the mother that keeps the uterus from contracting effectively) cannot be predicted in advance. We have no crystal ball; we only have the test of labor to give us the facts. If a baby simply cannot successfully pass through, the onus is finally off the mother to deliver vaginally. Every woman tries as hard as she can to have a vaginal delivery. If, say, after twenty hours of labor and two hours of unsuccessful pushing, she's completely wiped out and her baby's head cannot descend, she may need a cesarean. So be it. She shouldn't feel as though she has failed, or as though what awaits her is a surgical horror show.

• **Previous cesarean.** If a woman delivered her first baby by cesarean section, and the uterine incision was not the more common, side-to-side transverse incision, but instead a vertical or what is known as a classical incision, which cuts vertically through muscle, then she will automatically require a cesarean with any subsequent children. The vertical, or classical, incision puts a uterus at significant risk for rupture during a subsequent labor, so we would never deliver vaginally.

(For veterans only: If a woman has had a cesarean before, but isn't certain of the type of uterine incision she had, she ought to ask her doctor. A low transverse incision in the uterus makes a woman a candidate for an attempted vaginal delivery after cesarean [VDAC]. There is a less than one percent incidence of uterine rupture in the subsequent labors. For cosmetics and ease of healing, we usually perform transverse *skin* incisions, but don't think you can be certain of what type of uterine incision you had last time just by peering at the scar on your abdomen: There's no relationship between the skin incision and the uterine one.)

• **Previous Myomectomy.** This surgery for fibroid tumors may have weakened the uterine muscle, putting a woman at higher risk for uterine rupture. She will almost always be delivered by cesarean.

• **Baby's head cannot descend through the pelvis.** This includes very large (macrosomic) babies who, as I've mentioned earlier, have a different distribution of body fat, giving rise to the possibility of a crisis in delivery called shoulder dystocia, in which the baby's shoulders get "stuck." This can lead to palsy or paralysis of the arm. Large babies often don't descend through the birth canal even if the cervix becomes fully dilated. Cesarean section becomes the only option to accomplish delivery. The shape of a woman's pelvis may prevent even a normal-sized baby from descending.

• **Fetal distress.** When a fetal heartrate tracing is non-reassuring, or an abnormal scalp pH value confirms fetal distress, a C-section is done to reduce the risks of hypoxia (not enough oxygen) and associated cerebral palsy.

Cerebral palsy is classified as a motor disorder which leads to muscle spasms, paralysis, and, in 30 percent of all cases, mental retardation. CP is a poorly understood constellation of mental and physical developmental abnormalities. It's not entirely clear yet whether the development of the disorder is an antepartum (before delivery) or an intrapartum (during delivery) event. All of the modern technology that we now employ in childbirth has not seemed to reduce the risk of CP, which leads us to speculate it may in fact be an antepartum event. In other words, even though we're aggressive at diagnosing fetal distress in labor, we haven't cut down on the incidence of CP. That supports the idea that the disorder may occur long before the onset of the labor process, and it is not solely or at all the result of a birth trauma, but no one knows for sure.

• **Sudden, unexpected emergency.** Like pregnancy itself, most deliveries have unexpected moments and events that need to be watched closely or corrected—whether this involves a cord that briefly winds around a baby's neck, or a decelerated heartrate that might make it necessary for the mother to receive a dose of Terbutaline and some oxygen. But less common are the true medical emergencies—unexpected events that usually necessitate a fast cesarean. I want to emphasize that these are unusual situations, but even so, I will give you an example of two such unexpected emergencies that would cause a doctor to deliver by C-section:

   1. *Placental abruption.* Extremely rarely, the placenta will separate from the uterine wall sometime before delivery. This situation, called *abruptio placenta,* or placental abruption, disrupts the blood supply to the baby. It can be caused by hypertension, cocaine use, maternal trauma

such as a car accident, and certain diseases, such as lupus, that affect the maternal blood vessels.

2. *Prolapsed cord.* This is another relatively rare condition that sometimes happens when the membranes rupture, especially when the baby isn't head-down. A loop of umbilical cord actually drops into the vagina in front of the baby.

Once in the vagina it's compressed completely, so that blood can't flow through the cord, and the baby loses its source of oxygen. Delivery is considered an emergency situation, and a doctor might opt for a surgical rather than vaginal delivery, because delivery has to be accomplished quickly.

I had a patient who suddenly developed a prolapsed cord, and the scene was quite dramatic. In these situations, the doctor literally has to jump onto the bed with the mother and put her hand in the vagina, elevating the presenting part of the baby off the cord. My patient's bed was rushed down the hall into the operating room with the two of us in it, and the baby was delivered safely.

This rare situation can occasionally occur with a breech baby; sometimes, the baby's feet don't completely cover the cervix, and the cord drops down. Again, it's a true emergency, and very unlikely to happen to you.

THE PROCEDURE

There seems to be a feeling out there among patients that there's something a woman can do during her pregnancy to avoid having a C-section. *This is a myth*. Patients tell me they go religiously to exercise class, that they do hundreds upon hundreds of Kegel exercises, and that they are doing everything they can to get their pregnant bodies toned up for delivery. While it's wonderful to be in good physical condition for this demanding day and the ones that follow, in most cases fetal distress cannot be predicted, nor can certain complications be avoided.

Cesareans are usually performed using a regional anesthetic such as an epidural or a spinal. (The needle for a spinal is thinner than for an epidural, and penetrates the dura instead of the epidura, allowing for a one-time dose of long-lasting anesthetic that provides a denser, better block than an epidural.) General anesthesia is much more risky for pregnant women than for the rest of the population; there's a greater chance of aspirating contents of the stomach into the lungs, because of increased abdominal pressure and the relaxation of the lower esophagus, both side effects of pregnancy. There are some cases in which we have no choice but to use a general, but these are almost always emergencies, times when the baby simply must come out, and the woman doesn't have a functioning epidural in place.

Sometimes, when I make a decision to perform a cesarean, my patient becomes a bit freaked-out and squeamish, and begs me to knock her out completely, but I explain to her that it's far safer for her to be awake. I reassure her that her body will be appropriately draped, and that she won't see any of the surgery itself; she'll only see the baby as soon as it's born, which will be soon.

Here's how a cesarean is done: Say a woman has been in labor for twenty hours and she's totally wiped out. She hasn't eaten, she's barely slept, and all her attempts at pushing have failed. At this point, I will probably have a hasty heart-to-heart with her in which I let her know that I see how exhausted she is. I'll tell her that it seems cruel to make her go on like this, since statistically, if it was meant to be, it would have been already. After effective pushing for two to three hours, I can give her my opinion that it's time to proceed with a cesarean delivery. I try to ensure that she understands that I don't think she's being either "lazy" or "difficult" by not delivering vaginally, the way she had assumed she would.

Ultimately, whether or not to have a C-section is the patient's decision. If and when a woman has given consent, we thread a long, thin tube called a Foley catheter up into her bladder, in order to empty it of urine. This is important to do because a full bladder extends up into the operative field and could get injured during surgery. The top of the pubic hairline is then shaved. (Sorry.) Patients wince at the sight of the razor, but when the pubic hair grows back in, it entirely covers the incision, for which they're grateful.

At this point, we wheel the patient from the labor and delivery room into an available operating room. The O.R. is a dramatic change after spending so many hours in the relatively low-tech calm of a labor and delivery room. Now we achieve an adequate level of anesthesia. If she already has received an epidural (see page 182) a large dose of anesthetic is administered to numb the entire belly. We also give the patient some liquid antacid to neutralize the pH of the stomach contents; if she were to aspirate into her lungs, it wouldn't be as dangerous. (Acidic fluids, when aspirated, can severely damage the lungs, causing pneumonia and worse.) After the patient is given the antacid, she is positioned on the operating table. First we test to make sure she has enough anesthetic, by using a little pin to prick her skin. Once we are sure there's an adequate level for surgery, the doctor scrubs up with an assistant.

During a cesarean, there are always a handful of people around: the doctor; the assistant; the scrub nurse who hands the instruments to the doctors; the circulating nurse who walks around the room getting things; and, at the head of the table, the anesthesiologist. Pediatricians may or may not be called in. There's much more commotion in the O.R. than in the labor room; this doesn't mean something terrible is going on. Noise and commotion are to be expected.

The woman's belly will be prepped with Betadine, which is cold, but at this point she won't be able to feel the difference between cold or warm on her skin. She will just see someone painting the dark-brown liquid on her stomach, which will now feel removed from her body, since it has become totally devoid of sensation from the anesthetic.

Then the drape goes up and covers her field of vision. Her husband or birth partner will come and sit by her head. He's seated in a place where he isn't in the way of the doctors and nurses, and where he can comfort her. (He's allowed in the O.R. only if the woman is conscious; if we need to administer emergency general anesthesia and she'll be asleep during the operation, he's asked to leave.)

Then the surgery begins. The doctor makes an incision in the abdomen, usually what is known as a Pfannenstiel incision at the top of the hairline. After that first incision is made, the layers beneath the skin are methodically cut through, until the uterus is reached. Then an incision is made in the uterus itself—usually a "low transverse" incision. Many women seem to think that when a doctor cuts through the skin, he or she is also cutting so deeply that the uterus is cut into at the same time. That is not true; there are several layers in between. The incision that is made in the uterus may or may not be a transverse incision.

It takes about 30 to 40 minutes to perform a cesarean, but the baby is taken out in the first 5 or 10 minutes. For most women, the moment that she knows her baby is fine, the experience becomes much less overwhelming and frightening. After the baby has been delivered, a woman's energy is totally focused on the baby. But the doctors still have a good deal of work to do; on the other side of the drape, they need to carefully repair the layers of incisions they have made.

And now, a few words about my own cesarean. While I am quite reassuring to my patients who need the surgery done, I have to admit that I myself was petrified. I was $32^1/_2$ weeks pregnant, and I had preterm labor and premature rupture of membranes. By the time I was examined at the hospital I was already six centimeters dilated. The doctors weren't sure whether the twins' lungs were mature or not. So I was scared not only of the surgery but also of the outcome: What would my babies be like? They were premature; would they have long-lasting problems as a result? Everything was happening so fast, and I had no control over any of it. It's very hard for most people to give up control even in less dramatic situations, and during a cesarean that's exactly what you need to do. You become literally passive, your hands possibly restrained, your vision blocked. All this passivity is very different from the "activity" of labor. Things are happening to you in the operating room, yet you can't even feel them. And, to top it off, chances are that none of this has gone the way you had imagined it would. You'd imagined a perfect vaginal delivery. I felt that way, too, and now here I was, about to be "sectioned."

First I was given a spinal anesthetic, a one-shot deal with rapid onset. Within 30 seconds of the spinal being placed, I went completely numb from the waist down. I knew someone was moving my legs and inserting a Foley catheter, but I couldn't feel a thing. I felt as though the whole experience was happening to someone else, and I didn't have any sense of when they started cutting. Even though I was draped, I happened to notice that I had a good view of the goings-on in the reflecting glass of a medicine cabinet across the room. I could see Zack as he came out; I could even see him peeing on the doctor as she lifted him up. As the twins were born, I cried as easily and emotionally as my patients do. The rest of the cesarean took place as though in a dream; I was barely aware of any of it.

RECOVERY

Later, however, I was made *very* aware that it had happened, as are all women who have C-sections. It's a hard recovery, harder than I'd always counseled women it would be. I think having a cesarean has made me much more sympathetic and tolerant of my patients' postoperative complaints, as well as making me more lax about what a woman should be expected to do postoperatively. I used to march into patients' rooms on the morning after surgery (also called "Postoperative Day 1"), announcing that I wanted them to get out of bed, telling them that I knew it was going to be hard, but they really needed to get up and walk. Looking back now, I think there was something of an unfeelingly militaristic, no-nonsense style to these commands. In truth, I didn't quite understand the magnitude of what I was asking of them. When it came time for *me* to get up and walk after my cesarean, I found it almost unbearable.

I had been given a long-acting pain medication called Duramorph, which was administered directly into the spinal space. (This narcotic, and others like it, can be administered through an epidural, too.) The drugs are long-acting and help with postoperative pain control over the next 18 to 24 hours. They eliminate the need for calling for a nurse and waiting in pain for her to first bring the medication and then painstakingly prepare an injection. When the Duramorph wears off, a patient might be given some oral narcotic. Be aware, however, that all narcotics can create nausea, especially on an empty stomach.

Some women are given something called PCA, which stands for "patient-controlled anesthetic." This is an intravenous pump that the woman controls herself, administering as much or as little of the drug as she needs, and it can be enormously helpful.

Personally, I had a great deal of pain. I was surprised by how uncomfortable I was. The following morning, when the nurse removed my Foley catheter and I was free to get out of bed and go to the bathroom, I couldn't believe how hard it was to get all the way across the room. The bathroom seemed to be a million miles away; every step I took left me drenched with sweat. Once I got to the bathroom, my ordeal wasn't over by any means—I then had to find a way to sit down on the toilet, which seemed so low to the ground that it looked like a toilet in a preschool bathroom. It seemed that every step I took, every movement I made, was tearing my sutures open, ripping them apart.

By the time I got back to bed, I was totally exhausted, as though I had made an excursion to the top of the Statue of Liberty. I'd had visions of walking down to the special-care nursery to see the twins, but now I realized that I would need a wheelchair, which I continued to need for two days.

I now warn each C-section patient to expect the experience to be difficult in many ways. I tell her not to put Superwoman demands on herself now. If she needs a wheelchair to get around for a day or two, this isn't a tragedy.

Also as a result of my experience, one of the first things I tell women who have had cesareans is this: *You're going to think you're ripping open your incision, but you're not, and you can't.* Do yourself a favor and eliminate fear from the equation. It's the fear that holds you back as much as the pain. The pain can be managed with drugs, but the fear can be managed only through getting all the information and reassurance that you need.

The day of surgery is considered Day 0. The following day—Day 1—is when the urinary catheter will be taken out. The patient's diet is advanced now, too, either to clear liquids or more varied liquids. The intestines may not be ready for food yet, there's bound to be some nausea from the pain medications, and it's not a pleasant experience bringing up a plateful of spaghetti and meatballs.

Doctors look for signals to help them chart how the patient is progressing and when she can be started on solid food. An important indicator is that she's passed gas, which means her intestines are in working order. By Day 2, most patients are advancing to food. And by Day 3 or 4, they will probably be sent home.

Recovery from a cesarean is difficult not only because you've had abdominal surgery (which is always a tough recovery) but also because you're a mother now, and you'll be doing other things during your hospital stay, such as meeting with the pediatrician and perhaps breast-feeding or pumping milk. The whole issue of breast-feeding can seem overwhelming when you've just been through the ordeal of surgery, and if your early attempts at nursing don't go exactly as planned, you should know that you are hardly alone. Breast-feeding can be tricky in the beginning, and it seems more the rule than the exception that there will be some problems getting a routine established.

If a woman recovering from a C-section asks me if she can stay in the hospital until Day 5, I find myself in a tough position. The insurance companies consider that an excessive stay. If it were entirely up to me, I'd let her stay as long as she wants. (I know she could use it.) In the old days, women spent more time in the hospital after deliveries—both surgical and vaginal. I wish I could let patients stay in bed and rest until they really felt up to leaving. I wish, frankly, that the nurses and I could keep taking care of them, the way I wanted my nurses and my doctor to take care of me. But by the time these women are relatively mobile and functional and have graduated to solid foods, it's time for them to go home and get down to the business of motherhood.

Chapter Eleven
With Child

- In the Hospital
- Breast or Bottle
- Circumcision
- Homeward Bound
- Postpartum Depression
- When to Call the Doctor
- The Six-Week Visit
- Sex
- Slimming Down and Toning Up

One of the strangest experiences in life must be lying in a strange bed in a strange room in the middle of the night after giving birth, knowing that you are a mother. You've actually done it. After all these months of diligence, fear, excitement, and urine samples, it's happened. There's a baby either in your hospital room right now, or else in the nursery down the hall—someone with your name written on a bracelet attached to his or her wrist, as if the two of you are "going steady." And you are, in a way; the baby is yours, and you will need to learn how to take care of him or her. You will also, at the same time, need to learn how to take care of yourself. While your pregnant body came with a whole new set of rules to follow, so does your postpartum body.

IN THE HOSPITAL

As I said earlier, for the two nights you will most likely be in the hospital following a vaginal delivery (longer if you had a cesarean), you may well experience a certain degree of pain, which is normal. First of all, your uterus and vagina have gone through what is essentially a traumatic experience. Expect bleeding—a great deal of it, too—as the days go by. The fluid you pass is made up of blood and tissue from your uterus, which your body is getting rid of now that it no longer needs it. The bloody discharge is called lochia, and it will feel like the heaviest period of your life, but don't worry. The nurses will supply you with sanitary pads. Lochia may continue for up to six weeks, but with a significantly tapered flow.

Making matters even more unpleasant is the fact that you may well be recovering from an episiotomy. As I mentioned in Chapter 9, some women truly suffer from this incision, and the best way we know to treat the pain is with a combination of ice packs, cooling anesthetic spray, and Tylenol. Again, the nurses should provide you with everything you need, including a squeeze bottle and witch hazel pads; I find that ice packs are especially helpful for the first 24 hours, and you should keep one pressed against the very swollen vaginal region whenever you're lying in your hospital bed. Which leads me to remind you that you *should* be lying in bed now and taking it easy. Your entire body has been through one of the most intense physical experiences possible, and you will need to shore up your energy for days from now, when presumably you won't have an entire fleet of nurses waiting on you hand and foot.

Many women find themselves unable to urinate until several hours after delivery. Their bladders may have been temporarily affected by the pressure of a fetus, or by any anesthesia they received, or by the presence of a catheter. And if a woman is experiencing a great deal of pain and swelling in the perineum (and most women do) then urination can be quite painful. It's important that a woman urinates within roughly six to eight hours after delivery, to ensure that her bladder is functioning properly, and that she doesn't develop a bladder infection. (If you've ever had cystitis before—and most of us have—then you know how unpleasant it can be. Imagine experiencing cystitis *now*, on top of everything else.) If you continue to have trouble urinating, try the old "let-the-faucet-run" trick as a way of helping you get started. If hours pass and you still are unable, you should definitely ring for the nurse to discuss the matter further.

Bowel movements aren't quite as pressing—not yet, anyway. You'll need to have one eventually, but you'll know when that is. Women who have just delivered often live in mortal fear of the first postpartum bowel movement. It's similar to the anxieties women have when they're recovering from a cesarean: Those post-section women are scared to walk across a room for fear that they'll burst their stitches. Women who've had vaginal deliveries may be afraid to defecate because they fear they will burst their episiotomy stitches. All that straining, they figure, can't be good. They even think to themselves: Maybe I should just hold it in. . . .

Bad idea. The sooner that your body is back in working order—and that includes the rectum as well as the vagina—the better. One of the things I tell women recovering from a cesarean also applies here: *Eliminate fear from the equation. You will not rupture your incision.*

After a vaginal delivery, most hospitals routinely give women a stool softener; if you aren't offered one, you might want to request it. Usually the first bowel movement won't even happen until after you're home, but you can take the stool softener now.

Yet another discomfort that women experience after a vaginal delivery is something called afterpains. These are cramplike pains associated with the contractions of the uterus; they're a protective mechanism that helps decrease blood loss. When the placenta separates from the uterus after labor, huge blood vessels called sinuses open up, and now they all need to close. The uterus squeezes hard in order to compress these open sinuses. Afterpains don't tend to be severe in first-time mothers, but they can be quite painful with subsequent babies. Afterpains can often be felt most intensely when you're trying to nurse; as the baby pulls on the nipple, oxytocin (a hormone similar to Pitocin) is released, causing both the breast tissue and the uterus to contract. Tylenol and codeine derivatives can be given safely for afterpains even if you're nursing, so don't hesitate to ring for relief in the middle of the night. Nurses on the maternity floor expect patients to press their call buttons, and these nurses are kept busy bringing ice packs, Tylenol, and, once in a while, a baby from the nursery.

Which brings me to the question of where your baby will be sleeping. Most hospitals currently offer what is known as "rooming-in," which means the baby is allowed to spend the night with the mother, whether she's in a private room or not. In some places the father, however, can only spend the night if the mother has a private room. (These policies vary from hospital to hospital.) My patients tend to like rooming-in, because it allows them to start breast-feeding on the baby's—not the baby nursery's—schedule. But if you're really worn out from the delivery or in a tremendous amount of pain, then rooming-in may not be for you. Another option is a kind of modified rooming-in, in which you can have the baby with you for part of the night, then brought back to the nursery later, so that you can get some sleep. My feeling is that whatever arrangement you choose will be fine for your baby as well as for you. Your breast milk will not even be in yet, so your feeding sessions with your baby will serve only as a dress rehearsal. You will, however, have colostrum in your breasts, a yellowish pre-milk substance that you may have noticed in the weeks before the delivery, if you squeezed a nipple. Babies like colostrum, and, more importantly, they like and need to suck.

BREAST OR BOTTLE

These days, hospitals are competing with each other to offer a variety of services to new mothers. One extra frill they're concentrating on is the presence of an in-house lactation team—experts who will be able to help you get started breast-feeding before you and your baby go home. Some hospitals often maintain what's known as a "warm-line," which is a modified telephone hotline that can be called after you go home. The contact person can also put you in touch with a breast-feeding support group, which some women find helpful. Many places even make breast pumps available for purchase before you go home, and most will offer the use (or rental) of an electric pump during your stay if for some reason you can't breast-feed your baby but want to help your milk supply come in.

Hospitals want to be seen as "breast-feeding friendly," because there are often initiatives they're trying to meet, and accreditations they're trying to receive. In short, the reason that these services are offered may in fact be partly political, but you should certainly feel free to reap the benefits. If your hospital doesn't have any breast-feeding support built into the system, you do have other options. One obvious person to talk to is your pediatrician, who should be available to answer these and other ongoing questions. But another source of advice, at least in the beginning, is your obstetrician. While our hospital has plenty of in-house breast-feeding resources to offer its patients, I still field plenty of questions about getting started with nursing, and I'm always happy to answer them.

If you were to come to me after your baby is born and tell me how discouraged you were at your early attempts at breast-feeding, I would urge you not to feel bad and not to quit. Most new mothers have trouble establishing a good routine, and many of them tearfully threaten to stop before they've given it a full college try. But for more specific suggestions and tips, you might want to telephone the La Leche League, a national breast-feeding advocacy organization that has branches throughout the country. While a number of its members seem to take a hard-line view that breast-feeding is the only way to go, as a whole the organization does some very good work. After you get home from the hospital, you can look up the La Leche League in your local phone book and be able to speak to someone 24 hours a day. These women firmly believe in the practice of nursing, and they are eager to help first-time mothers.

Breast-feeding has been proven to be best for babies, helping to boost their immune systems and preventing them from experiencing milk allergies and constipation. No one knows how many months a baby needs to nurse in order to receive the optimum immunity and health benefits, but I quote to my patients the World Health Organization's claims that a full six months of nursing is ideal. Breast-feeding also serves as a natural form of birth control (though not to a fully reliable degree; sorry, you'll still need to use some other kind of contraception, too).

I nursed Samantha and Zachary for four weeks (which, with twins, felt like four months), and I'm glad I did. There's a tremendous feeling of accomplishment to be had in nursing: It's as though you can't really believe that your body can fully nourish another living person. (Or, in my case, two living persons.) Breast-feeding also lets you travel light: no bottles, no nipple brushes, no formula—just you, your breasts, and your baby.

But every woman's lifestyle is different. Maybe you're eager to get back to work and don't want the hassle of pumping breast milk every day. Maybe you simply don't like the physical notion of breast-feeding. Maybe the pregnancy really knocked the wind out of your sails and you want to reclaim your body now. Maybe you have other children at home who need your attention. It's up to you; I would never be doctrinaire about such a personal decision. But like your mother probably used to say to you when she wanted you to eat your vegetables: Just try it. And if you don't like it, at least you can say you gave it a chance.

Sometimes barriers arise even for women who are determined to breast-feed. Intermittent clogged ducts are common, a condition in which the normal secretion of milk is blocked. The treatment for this is to continue breast-feeding, massage the affected breast, and apply warmth. Occasionally a clogged duct can turn into mastitis, an infection of the breast that is usually bacterial in origin. The symptoms of mastitis are fever (sometimes as high as 104°), redness, and swelling. The infection is usually treated with antibiotics, and women are encouraged to continue nursing if possible, or to use a pump if the baby can't latch onto the nipple due to the changed shape of the areola.

Sometimes renting or buying a breast pump is a good idea, especially for women who have to return to work quickly or are experiencing problems with the baby latching on. The advantage is that even if the baby has to drink from a bottle, the bottle at least contains breast milk.

I know of doctors who try to coax all their patients to breast-feed. I generally tell women that breast-feeding offers several advantages, but that formula does not offer disadvantages. If, however, you know for a fact that you won't be breast-feeding, you will probably be instructed to let the milk dry up in your breasts without the aid of medications. In the past, women were given a drug called Parlodel (bromocriptine), which suppresses lactation, but because of side effects, it's no longer FDA-approved for this use. So if you're looking for the quick fix that your Mom received, sorry, it doesn't exist anymore.

When a woman's not planning to breast-feed, I instruct her to bind her breasts as much as possible. She should wear a tight, supportive bra (sports bras are good) so that her breasts receive minimal stimulation. Breasts are incredibly easily confused; they're sort of a "stupid" organ, in that even walking around and having your nipples rub against the nightgown could be construed by your breasts as a baby trying to nurse, and thereby provide a stimulus to produce milk.

If, on day three after delivery, you become engorged—which means your breasts fill up and become rock-hard and extremely painful—ice packs and pain medications are the appropriate treatment. Most women, unless they've had a cesarean or some complication, are already home by the time engorgement occurs. Some women even develop a fever associated with engorgement, which ought to be mentioned to the doctor. Most likely, though, you'll only have one difficult day at the most.

The breasts may be stupid in some ways, but in other ways they're also incredibly smart; they work beautifully within a system of supply and demand, creating more milk when it's necessary, and eventually ceasing production of milk when no one's there to drink it.

CIRCUMCISION

New mothers and fathers often are at a loss as to whether or not to circumcise their newborn sons. If they aren't adhering to any religious or cultural dictates, then the decision may be even more difficult to make. Medical experts go back and forth as to the medical relevance of the procedure, which involves the surgical removal of the foreskin of the penis.

One factor that might help new parents make the decision is whether or not the baby's father is circumcised. It's useful for a boy, in terms of gender identification, to have a penis that "looks like Daddy's." Also, the latest medical thinking has shown that circumcision leads to a decreased risk of both urinary tract infections and long-term penile cancers. Some of these cancers start with a virus that can occur in the absence of good enough hygiene; it's much more difficult to clean an uncircumcised penis, because bacteria can collect under the foreskin. Relatedly, uncircumcised men seem to have a greater chance of passing these viruses on to their female sexual partners; some tentative links have been established between uncircumcised men and cervical cancers in women.

But these findings may be challenged in the future, and the pendulum may in fact swing the other way soon enough. Already in the United States, as has been the case in Europe for a long time, many parents are choosing not to have their sons circumcised. If a woman and her partner remain undecided, then I suggest that they speak with their pediatrician.

But if they want my opinion (and do perform the circumcision on some babies the morning after their birth), then I am happy to give it to them. In most cases, I tell them, I think circumcision is a good idea.

HOMEWARD BOUND

Once you've gotten the okay from your doctor to leave the hospital (and, believe me, your insurance company really wants your doctor to release you), then it's time to return home. If you've had a vaginal delivery, your doctor will have given you some basic instructions for taking care of the vaginal region and any sutures. You will be sent off with your plastic squeeze-bottle and perhaps with a prescription for a mild pain reliever, such as Tylenol with codeine.

He or she will also instruct you not to take a bath or go swimming for the next six weeks, whether you've had a vaginal delivery or a C-section. The theory behind this is that your body hasn't reestablished its mucous plug, which provides the barrier that keeps your uterus a sterile environment. The endometrium, which is the lining of the uterus, is a sterile place. It's an impressive system that needs more time to get back in working order, and before that happens, you should not let water enter it.

Nor should you insert anything in your vagina for six weeks, either, whether it's a tampon or a penis. I tell women: "No swimming, no douching, no intercourse"—and they say, "No *problem*." For most women, all of these acts are completely unappealing right now; they've got a baby to take care of, they've had no sleep, and, besides, they're bleeding continuously.

Armed with a set of instructions and a baby, new mothers venture out into the world, which can suddenly seem like a different place than when they left it just a couple of days ago. While the hospital can be a difficult, exhausting experience, sometimes a kind of fear sets in upon leaving this place. Now you're really on your own—you and your new family.

Besides which, another realization may occur to you as you enter life with a newborn in your arms; just as it seemed almost incredible, close to nine months earlier, to think that you were actually pregnant, it may seem equally incredible now to think that you're not. It may, in fact, seem sad. You may start to miss how special you felt, the way people looked at you a certain way on the street, or always gave up their seat on a bus (well, perhaps *occasionally* gave up their seat, at least in New York City). Of course, you will be showered with extra attention as you hit the streets and the buses with your new baby in tow, but it won't be quite the same. Being pregnant can feel like a wonderful secret that's slowly shared with the world as the baby grows inside you and becomes an unmistakable reality. *Not* being pregnant anymore is startling; the state of pregnancy is so intense and involving that while you're pregnant you may almost forget that it will one day end.

POSTPARTUM DEPRESSION

A combination of wistfulness, hormones, overwork, and fatigue serves to create what we unofficially call the postpartum blues. Giving birth to a child and then becoming responsible for him or her day and night is an enormous, dramatic burden, and it tends to wear down the body's mechanisms. Seventy to 80 percent of all women who've just had babies experience some form of the blues. Most of my patients find themselves bursting into tears for no good reason at least once, or feeling irritable and bitterly arguing with their spouses over such major issues as whose turn it is to change a diaper. There may be a sense that having a baby was a mistake. There's a good chance that a woman in the midst of postpartum blues will feel lonely and isolated, as though she will never get her "real life" back. She may also feel overrun, especially if she has a baby nurse living with her—a total stranger who seems to know a lot more about baby care than *she* does. Sometimes, if a woman's mother comes to help out after the baby arrives, certain tensions can arise, and certain old problems in the relationship between mother and daughter are reactivated. The mother may insist that she's "just trying to help," but her distraught daughter may feel criticized, bossed around, and just plain miserable, so much so that she may disappear into the linen closet for the occasional good cry.

All of these postpartum scenarios are totally normal. I experienced a couple of them myself. Because Samantha and Zachary were premature, they had to stay in the hospital longer than I did. I'd had an image of Jeff and myself leaving the hospital with two bundles in our arms, and not being able to do that was upsetting. I was tearful for several days when I went to visit them in the nursery. There they were, lying in their isolettes: perfect, helpless, yet strong. The beauty of it all—and the frustration—made me burst quietly into tears.

We've all had moments when a sudden flood of emotion threatens to overwhelm us. And then, for most of us, those moments pass. What distinguishes the postpartum blues from true postpartum depression (which is a much more serious situation, and is actually classified as an illness) is severity, as well as persistence of symptoms. It's difficult to make an accurate diagnosis of postpartum depression, given how prevalent the more common blues can be right now.

When a woman comes to me for a six-week appointment, in addition to performing a physical exam I'll also try to give her the once-over with regard to her emotional state. Of course, this is tough to do in a twenty-minute office visit, but some details might raise a red flag for me, such as excessive tearfulness, and a heightened emotional state as we talk. Her degree of grooming can give me a sense of how well she's taking care of herself; depressed mothers often have a hard time managing to comb their hair or take a shower. If she's brought the baby with her, as I peek into the carriage and coo and compliment, I'll make sure the baby looks clean and well-cared-for, too.

I once had a patient who became convinced, in the hospital, that the nurses were manhandling her baby. She tearfully told me, "They throw my baby around in the nursery. I can't believe they treat him like this." I knew that the nursing staff was gentle and competent, and I felt my patient's view was untrue, a distortion. Her response did not seem normal to me, and I had someone come down from Psychiatry to talk to her and make sure it was safe to release her. In the end she turned out to be fine, but I needed to make sure. In its most dramatic (but rare) forms, postpartum depression can develop into actual psychosis, in which women are at risk of harming themselves or their babies.

One of the problems with dealing with postpartum depression is that even in this age of supposed openness, many people still attach a stigma to any symptoms that can be classified as mental—as opposed to physical—illness. Some of my patients feel that they're weak if they experience any emotional vulnerability, or if they dare to admit it to anyone. I try to assure them that a certain degree of emotional vulnerability or difficulty after childbirth is to be expected, and that even when the difficulty becomes excessive and warrants the help of a therapist, it doesn't mean they are "bad" or "weak" mothers.

The Superwoman syndrome can play an insidious role here; recently a patient admitted to me that she'd been depressed for five months after the birth of her baby. I was astonished. "Why didn't you call me?" I asked. "I was embarrassed," she said. I knew that if she'd had any physical complaints—pain or bleeding or an infection of any kind—she wouldn't have hesitated to pick up the telephone. But because her distress was emotional, she felt ashamed.

Obstetricians are very sympathetic to the problems of new

mothers, and this includes problems that may, in the long run, be outside our province, such as psychiatric concerns. But we want to know if a patient is experiencing distress so that we can help direct her toward the help she needs. Postpartum depression responds well to certain psychiatric drugs and sometimes to therapy; if you are experiencing more than your share of distress, you should definitely inform your doctor.

WHEN TO CALL THE DOCTOR

In addition to postpartum depression, there are other conditions that warrant a telephone call to your doctor before the six-week visit. They include:

• **Excessive bleeding.** As I mentioned at the start of this chapter, heavy bleeding following delivery is completely normal. But many women want to know exactly how much blood is too much, and I have to say that it's hard to quantify. Excessive blood loss is associated with women who carried twins or triplets, because the uterus is so stretched out that it has difficulty contracting well. Excessive blood loss may also be due to retained fragments of placenta, or an unrecognized laceration in the vagina. While some doctors take the number of sanitary pads that a woman soaks through in a given amount of time as an indication of whether the bleeding is excessive, I don't find this very useful, since some women may change pads before they're completely soaked through.

In the hospital, the nurses take note of a patient's blood loss, but when she returns home she'll need to do that for herself. If bleeding suddenly increases after the first two days, she ought to contact her doctor. (This goes for a woman who's had a cesarean, too, although typically she will bleed for less time—two to three weeks—due to a more effective cleaning-out of her uterus at the time of delivery.)

Usually, bleeding tapers off into "nuisance" bleeding for the next four to six weeks, but if it doesn't, or if it remains continuous and unrelentingly heavy, or increases dramatically, this is considered excessive. You should call your doctor if you feel lightheaded or faint.

If your discharge is foul-smelling, or if you develop an unexplained fever above 100.4°, you ought to speak with your doctor. Other reasons to call are:

• Red, swollen, painful breasts.

• Pinpoint pain at the episiotomy site.

• Burning on urination.

If something is bothering you physically in the time period between leaving the hospital and going in for the six-week visit, you shouldn't hesitate to call your doctor; infections and other complications do occasionally occur, and they may need to be treated.

THE SIX-WEEK VISIT

This appointment takes place at an essentially arbitrary amount of time after giving birth. Six weeks isn't a magic number, although by this point the uterus has been allowed to return to its normal size (about as big as a pear), bleeding has resolved, the episiotomy has healed, and, if a woman has had a cesarean, that scar has healed as well. If there have been any problems in the interim, such as heavy bleeding that continues after the first month, or continued pain and fever signaling an infection, I should have already heard from the patient.

At the six-week appointment, I can pretty much assess the state of a woman's pelvic recovery by the way she walks into the office—whether her movements are normal or whether, in the rare case, she still has that "saddle-sore" look that women have after they've just given birth. I perform a pelvic exam to ensure that everything has healed well and has returned to its prepregnancy state. I also do a Pap smear, breast exam, and thyroid exam (sometimes thyroid problems develop after a pregnancy), and I initiate a discussion about birth control.

SEX

When I mention the subject of birth control, some women look at me as if I'm crazy. "Do you really think I'm interested in ever having sex again?" they say. But I tell them that, believe it or not, they may in fact feel like having sex again sometime soon, and they ought to be prepared. If their method of birth control is the diaphragm, they will need to be refitted, because no doubt the delivery has changed them internally. If they used to take the Pill but they're still nursing, I'm really not comfortable starting them back on it yet. Some hormonal methods of birth control are considered safe for nursing mothers by other doctors, but I just don't think a baby ought to be ingesting these powerful chemicals through its mother's milk. I would recommend, instead, that women who are used to taking the Pill switch to a diaphragm or condom and spermicide until they've stopped nursing.

Most of my patients are afraid that intercourse will hurt, and they're right. It does hurt at first, perhaps more than it did the first time they ever had sex. The vagina has gone through a great ordeal, and the episiotomy stitches (if there are any) will have tightened the vagina, so that it now has less "give." A water-based lubricant such as K-Y jelly can help, especially if a woman is nursing; the hormones of nursing keep the vagina less lubricated than normal.

But the only way to completely stop sex from hurting is by getting back into the swing of it slowly—in essence, continuing to attempt to have intercourse even when it doesn't feel like the most pleasurable act in the world. One day, you will enjoy it again. (And maybe one day, the baby will actually sleep through the night, so that you and your partner can have a little uninterrupted time in bed.)

SLIMMING DOWN AND TONING UP

If lack of interest in sex lasts for a month or two after the pain of intercourse has passed, this may well indicate a psychological component. I'm not a psychiatrist, but I would venture an opinion that sometimes women can feel self-conscious about their bodies after giving birth, especially if they haven't returned to their prepregnancy weight. And that brings me to the topic of weight loss after delivery, which can be either the easiest thing in the world to accomplish, or the bane of your existence.

Sometimes a patient comes to see me at six weeks and she's already shed all her extra weight. Other times a woman comes to the office and says she still has 20 pounds to go. It's extremely variable. I strongly feel that, like so many other things in life, how quickly you will snap back to your prepregnancy body is determined partly by luck and partly by genes. The pregnancy has redistributed your weight, centering it on the hips and the belly now. Getting rid of it in these places takes concentrated, targeted exercise. By six weeks, you'll certainly be permitted to exercise, and you're welcome to do abdominals, too, in order to tone this area that has been so greatly softened and loosened by pregnancy. Although I don't recommend Kegel exercises during pregnancy, I do strongly recommend doing them postpartum in order to tighten the vaginal muscles. This will also keep down the incidence of occasional "incontinence" that sometimes continues to happen once in a while after childbirth, just as it did occasionally during pregnancy.

I recommend joining a postpartum exercise class at a local Y or gym, which can give women the opportunity to get fit through a workout specifically designed to combat the wear and tear of pregnancy on such areas as the stomach and lower back. Some of these classes allow new mothers to bring their babies with them; when the babies are very little, they can often be worked into some of the exercise routines. If actually getting out of the house and making it all the way to a class seems daunting, there are a variety of postpartum exercise videos on the market, most of which have the same emphases. And then there's the exercise that new mothers will get simply from walking a baby carriage or stroller down the street. Women often aren't aware of how much mileage they're clocking when they're with their infants, but it may be a surprising amount. Remembering to keep the pace brisk can turn a simple stroll into an aerobic boost.

But it's all completely up to you. While you were pregnant, issues such as weight and exercise were of major concern both to you and your obstetrician; now your doctor may offer suggestions and specific diet and exercise advice and encouragement, but for the most part you're really on your own. You've gone through an entire pregnancy and come out the other side—intact and beaming and encumbered by a heavy diaper bag—oh, and, yes, a baby.

I sometimes feel a slight twinge when my work with a patient is through; after all, I've gotten to know her pretty well over the months, and now we won't be seeing each other on a regular basis. But more to the point, I usually feel a real sense of satisfaction from having led her through her entire pregnancy and delivered her baby safely.

Many women bring their newborns to the six-week visit, or at least bring photos of them to put in our extremely thick office brag book. Babies are worth bragging about, of course; each one is amazing and tender and unique, and no matter how many I deliver in my lifetime, I imagine I will always feel this way. But it seems to me that mothers deserve their own brag book, too, a document of everything they went through to help this baby develop: all the jumbo vitamins they swallowed and the tests they endured, all the times they climbed onto the scale or hoisted themselves onto the table. In short, all the attention they paid and the discomfort they experienced—all the aches both large and small.

But it still amazes me how quickly the aches of pregnancy fade, how eventually they begin to recede after the fact. That happened to me, too, despite all the information I'd gathered during my medical training and during my own nine months. Childbirth is a great equalizer; whether or not you've also been through the rigors of an obstetrical residency, there's nothing like the sight and feel and smell of a new baby to make all the worries and the endless details you've been obsessing over fly out the window forever. In their place is a wonderful new person (whom you'll eventually worry about and obsess over, too). But for now, in the early weeks and months of motherhood, I urge you to keep life simple and to accept any offers of help that come your way, so you can spend enough time enjoying the multitude of pleasures and surprises that your baby brings. Doctor's orders.

INDEX

abdominal wall defects, 101

abortion, 95

abruptio placenta, 43, 84, 207

Accutane, 79

acetaminophen, 78

aches, *see* pains and aches

acne treatments, 79, 80

AFP (alphafetoprotein), 100–101, 102, 103, 104
  maternal serum, 101, 102–3, 104, 105

afterbirth, 199–200

alcohol, 76–77, 82, 110

AMA (advanced maternal age), 107

amniocentesis, 98, 103, 104, 105–10
  CVS vs., 38, 39
  doctor's experience in, 109
  inaccuracies in, 106
  ultrasound in, 106–7
  whether to have, 94–97, 103

amniotic fluid, 140, 146

amniotic sac (membranes), rupturing of, 105, 166–69, 172, 176, 181

amniotomy, 181

anemia, 148–49
  sickle-cell, 35, 36, 39
  thalassemia, 35

anencephaly, 99, 101

anesthesia:
  in cesareans, 209, 210–11
  epidural, *see* epidural
  general, 183, 209, 211
  patient-controlled, 214
  spinal, 209, 213

anesthesia staff, 8

ankles, 114, 115

antibiotics, 80

antidepressants, 80–82

Apgar scores, 199

artificial sweeteners, 74

Ashkenazic triple-screen, 35, 36

aspirin, 78

asthma, 43–44

baby, 197–99, 200–201, 227–28, 236–37
  Apgar scores of, 199
  breast-feeding of, *see* breast-feeding
  circumcision of, 225–26
  low birth weight in, 75–76
  macrosomic, 61–62, 146, 206
  physical appearance of, 197–98
  rooming-in at hospital, 220–21
  see also fetus